Order this book online at www.trafford.com/08-0495
or email orders@trafford.com

Most Trafford titles are also available at major online book retailers.

Note for Librarians: A cataloguing record for this book is available from Library and Archives Canada at www.collectionscanada.ca/amicus/index-e.html

ISBN: 978-1-4251-7627-3

We at Trafford believe that it is the responsibility of us all, as both individuals and corporations, to make choices that are environmentally and socially sound. You, in turn, are supporting this responsible conduct each time you purchase a Trafford book, or make use of our publishing services. To find out how you are helping, please visit www.trafford.com/responsiblepublishing.html

Our mission is to efficiently provide the world's finest, most comprehensive book publishing service, enabling every author to experience success. To find out how to publish your book, your way, and have it available worldwide, visit us online at www.trafford.com/10510

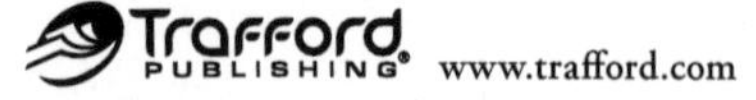

www.trafford.com

North America & international
toll-free: 1 888 232 4444 (USA & Canada)
phone: 250 383 6864 • fax: 250 383 6804 • email: info@trafford.com

The United Kingdom & Europe
phone: +44 (0)1865 722 113 • local rate: 0845 230 9601
facsimile: +44 (0)1865 722 868 • email: info.uk@trafford.com

10 9 8 7 6 5 4 3 2

Prologue

The Health For Life book is a practical work and the product of many years of prayer, study, research and life experience in walking with God. It is written for anyone who has an interest in health, healing and a desire to understand what the bible has to say about health and how to apply it in their lives. It is also written for those who want to develop further in these areas and discover more about the journey of biblical wholeness. There are scriptural examples, references, practical guidelines, chapter summaries, reflective questions and testimonies in addition to a biblical basis and scientific accuracy. As a medical practitioner and Christian minister, I am for biblical accuracy and scientific fact. I trust that you will find this book integrating the two in a clear, non jargon way that gives glory to God. Its purpose is not to provide a comprehensive theological or scientific work but rather to provoke thought, provide guidance and activate action in a vitally important and fascinating area of life and godliness.

The health care arena is influenced by many models of health belief. Conventional medicine historically has been influenced by Greek philosophy, principles and deities. The Hippocratic Oath formed the basis of early medical ethics. Eastern philosophy, New Age beliefs and ancient arts of healing are now competing against this traditional model of western health care. Whilst appreciating the advancements some of these models have made, I ultimately believe that the Judeo Christian model of health is the truest reflection of who we are as people.

In approaching this topic it is critical to understand that biblical health is a grace issue founded upon our relationship with God. Faith in Jesus Christ grants us status as children of God. This is not conditional upon our good works and human effort. From this place of security and rest we find spiritual fulfilment. This can produce peace of mind, wholesome relationships, stable emotions and healthy life choices. All these factors impact upon our physical well being.

Many people attempt to find spiritual fulfilment and healthy relationships through physical well being. Whilst physical health can enhance our spiritual and relational condition it does not satisfy the deepest human needs. Hence an *integrated* approach to health care must address the framework of the whole person in a spirit, soul, and body order.

The opinions and values held in this book are my personal beliefs based upon my understanding of scripture, life experience and medical practice. In reading and reflecting upon its content I hope that you will find the pathway to biblical wholeness.

Dr Liam Chapman

Dedications and Acknowledgements

This book is dedicated firstly to Jesus Christ whose love we can never fully comprehend. The depth of what He did in my life and family I cannot express in words but only in gratitude to Him. Secondly, it is dedicated to all those people who will come to faith in Christ because of it. Eternal destiny is far too important to relegate to the death bed. Thirdly, it is dedicated to all those people who will find encouragement, hope, restoration and purpose as a result of it. Your life was meant for living and God gave it as a gift for you to enjoy as well as endure.

In producing this book there are many people to acknowledge:

Rev Wynne Lewis, my first Pastor in Kensington Temple, London.
Rev Colin Dye, his successor, under whose ministry I had opportunity to grow, develop and serve an apprenticeship in the ministry. His heart for the healing ministry and personal concern was a catalyst to an apostolic vision for revival and reform.
Rev Dr Michael Carr, my present Pastor at Harrow International Christian Centre. His wisdom, insight, maturity and straightforwardness have refined my character, maturity and wholeness in life and ministry.
Rev Roger Stedman, who has been a faithful friend and minister over many years. Rev Alistair Taylor, who provided an initial springboard for me to speak on biblical health and Rev Geoffrey Blease, who has sought to bring this to a wider audience.

A special acknowledgement goes to my spiritual parents Constant and Jennifer Kwitegetse from Uganda. They brought me to Christ in 1988 and have been a constant source of love, encouragement and nurture over the years. Their love has been unconditional and ministry consistent through decades of commitment to the cause of Christ.

The many hundreds of friends, partners, ministers, believers and colleagues, who have influenced my life, prayed for me and strengthened my faith.
Mr Bradley Loubser who has shared this journey with me over the past 10 years and formatted this book to the quality you see today.

My parents, brother, sisters and in laws who have loved, accepted, and encouraged me through the years in all that I have done. Your love and relationship is priceless to me.

Most importantly, my dear wife Jean who I love immeasurably and trust unreservedly. She is my soul mate and my life partner. My children, Daniel and Elisha who make me proud to be a father.

About the author

Dr Liam Chapman

Liam was born in Yorkshire and grew up in Silsden, West Yorkshire within walking distance of beautiful countryside. His mother originated from Cheshire and his father from Dublin. He is the grandson of a lay Methodist preacher. He is proud of his Yorkshire roots and values the frank honesty and simplicity of its life and values. He was inspired towards Medical Missions after reading 'Mister Leprosy' by Phyllis Thompson (ISBN: 0340258373) in his teenage years. In 1988 he came to London to study medicine and stayed at the Alliance Club belonging to the China Inland Mission (missionary organisation of Hudson Taylor, the pioneering missionary to China). Within three weeks he had made a definite commitment to Christ.

Over the next 14 years he attended Kensington Temple, London, and was involved in evangelism, missions, pastoral leadership of cell groups and churches. He qualified in medicine in 1993 (MBBS), General Practice specialisation in 2004 (MRCGP) and Tropical Medicine and Hygiene in 1995 (DTM&H).

1998 was a turning point in his life and ministry. God laid on his heart a desire for revival and reform in the nations including missions, health and the church. In 2000 he founded a missionary organisation based in northern Uganda, The East African Missionary Society. In 2001 he launched the Centre of Integrated Medicine (CIM). The heart of this ministry is to see the revelation and realisation of the reality of 'Christ In Me' as spirit, soul and body people. This included a biblical health medical practice, health consultancy for ministers, research and proclamation of the biblical health message through public speaking, literature, media and audiovisual.

This culminated in the founding of 'Partners In Ministry' in 2004 as an umbrella charity for the ministry. It also brings together the wider ministry to local churches, ministries and organisations in Britain and the nations.

Since 2002 he has been an active member of Harrow International Christian Centre where he is an associate minister and missions director.

He is happily married to Jean who has shared many of the ministry responsibilities with him. She is a nurse in General Practice and they have two children, Daniel and Elisha.

Introduction

Health is a multi-million pound global enterprise. To some it represents an exercise regime, to some a constant reminder of their lack of it. For others it is a reaction to 21st century living and lifestyle or perhaps even a whole belief system affecting their way of life. Biblical health is more than all of these. It encompasses spiritual, emotional and relational life as well as physical well-being. Global trends are bringing issues of health to the central agenda. These include globalization, urbanization, westernisation, ageing populations, increasing population densities, environmental concerns, nutritional issues, traditional values and community fragmentation. From the industrial revolution through the age of exploration, scientific enlightenment and the information technology age we now live in a global village with great benefits but also tremendous challenges.

Consequences and challenges we face physically as humans are the following:

1. Growing 'older iller' due to the increase in chronic diseases like diabetes and heart disease. Chronic disease management is rapidly becoming the medicine of the 21st century
2. A resurgence of infectious diseases like tuberculosis
3. 'New' viruses such as HIV, SARS, Avian Flu
4. The threat of environmental toxicity with nuclear, GM, intensive farming and climate change

Divorce, fatherless ness, abuse of various kinds, Internet pornography and a diversity of mental illnesses have ravaged our marriages, families and communities both personally and relationally.

Spiritually our societies are in a huge cultural transition. Post modern, post enlightenment, secularism and multi-culturism are now part of our identity as a society and nation. The very foundation of our society as a Christian nation is being challenged and changed.

I have highlighted the true, yet seemingly negative, aspects of modern health status. This is to emphasise the huge potential there is for churches, leaders, ministries and individuals to respond positively with the definitive answers the bible provides. The fundamental issues of need have not changed since the Garden of Eden but the complexities and rate of change have.

People still desire:

Spiritual fulfilment
Emotional stability and security
Social communities
Relational completeness
Physical vitality and well-being

Faiths, complementary and alternative therapies, science and secularism continue to grapple to provide the answers. The world, the flesh and the devil have not changed in desire, purpose or operation. Jesus understood in creation that God gave us His *Ruach* (spirit) to become a *nephesh* (living soul) in a *soma* (body) with a garden. Biblical health brings together who we are, where we are, what we are and why we are. With these answers God can have a voice through His people that brings a message of restoration and wholeness to the church. It is one of the few means by which the church can communicate the gospel to the world in a language they can understand and meet a need they know they have.

CONTENTS

SECTION ONE - BACKGROUND

CHAPTER ONE
BIBLICAL BASIS

A. IS HEALTH BIBLICAL?

This first section is somewhat foundational but necessary for a basic understanding to the topic as a whole and will help to put the remainder in context. There are two questions to answer here:

Is health a biblical word and concept?
Is being biblical healthy?

To answer the first we need to look at what health is and if the bible speaks about that. In answering the second we need to review the response to the first question and see if an 'evangelical' Christian who believes the bible to be true, representative and accurate is in a healthy state themselves. I will look in depth at the general meaning of the word health in Part B - Healing vs. Health, but here are some of the biblical meanings and scriptural references.

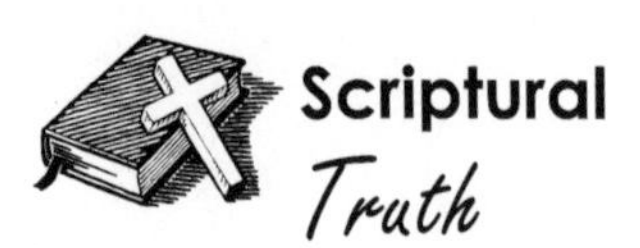

1. To lengthen/prolong – *arukah* (Hebrew)

Isaiah 58:8 – 'Thine health shall spring forth speedily'
Jeremiah 30:17 – 'I will restore health unto thee'
Jeremiah 33:6 – 'I will bring it health and cure'

2. Safety and security – *yeshuah* (Hebrew)

Psalms 42:1; Psalms 43:5 – 'Who is the health of my countenance'

3. Completeness of healing – *marpe* (Hebrew)

Proverbs 4:22 – 'Health to all their flesh'
Proverbs 12:18 – 'But the tongue of the wise is health'
Proverbs 13:17 – 'But a faithful ambassador is health'

Jeremiah 8:15 – 'For a time of health'

4. **Physical healing – *riphuth* (Hebrew)**

   Proverbs 3:8 – 'It shall be health to thy navel'

5. **Peace, completeness – *shalom* (Hebrew)**

   2 Samuel 20:9 - 'Are you in health my brother?'

6. **Soundness – *soteria* (Greek)**

   Acts 27:34 – 'Take some meat for your health'

7. **State of being – *hygiaino* (Greek)**

   3 John 2 – 'That you may prosper in all things and be in health'

From the following it is clear that the concept of biblical health is more than divine healing and miracles. It includes:

- **Preservation, prolongation and longevity.**
- **Wholeness that involves our whole being, how we speak, our relationships and times and seasons of our lives.**
- **Physical healing**
- **Peace**
- **Balance and soundness**
- **A state of being**

Biblical health takes us beyond merely focusing on the physical into our state of being as a whole and how that interacts with God, relationships and the world around us.

It is a place of balance and not for the fitness fanatics only. It has sound scientific and knowledge principles. It begins with our identity in Christ (spiritual health) and not a state of 'doing' where we strive in our own strength. It is a place of rest and not condemnation or guilt because of our present lack of health.

To answer the second question we need to reflect on ourselves and think about fundamental issues that include our identity, security, role and purpose (see 'Reflective Time', pg 15).

Initially at this stage it is good to answer those questions at a fairly 'gut' level response. Later you can do this in greater detail when we look at spiritual health.

Conclusion

In concluding this introduction to 'Is health biblical?' it is important to emphasise that because biblical health encompasses such a wide area of our lives, we are all on the journey into health. We are not fully complete or in health until we take on our eternal state in glory. Because we still have issues does not mean we are not 'biblical'.

My second question is simply to promote reflection and pursue personal, physical, relational and ministerial development. Because you're not healthy right now doesn't mean that you are not a bible believing Christian! God's purpose 'in health' I believe, is simply that we should aim to be 'all that He wants us to be in every area of our lives.'

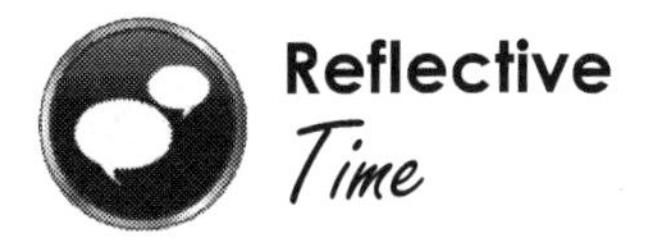

1. **Who am I? – identity**
2. **Where am I? – security**
3. **What am I? – role**
4. **Why am I? – purpose**

Personal *Thoughts*

B. HEALING VERSUS HEALTH

There are three important concepts to distinguish:

1. Healing (divine or biblical)

This encompasses restoration of the body (and sometimes the mind or emotions) to its natural and correct function. It is a restoration of what was lost or a repair of what was broken. An analogy is of a car that has a flat tyre, which is repaired to its former state. Healing can include medicine or healing remedies and a sense of wholeness as well as prayer and the laying on of hands. There is a link or progression toward health in certain meanings of the word 'heal':

- To repair – *rapha* (Hebrew)
  Genesis 20:17 – 'God healed Abimelech'
- To attend to – *therapeuo* (Greek) – as in therapy or therapeutics
  Matthew 4:23 – 'healing all manner of sickness'
- To plan or intent – *eis iasis* (Greek)
  Acts 4:30 – 'by stretching forth Thine hand to heal'
- Absolute (and often immediate) – *iaomai* (Greek)
  Matthew 8:8 – 'Speak the word only and my servant shall be healed'
- Supernatural – *iama* (Greek)
  1 Corinthians 12:9 – 'The gifts of healing'
- Soundness, wholeness – *sozo* (Greek)
  Luke 8:36 – 'possessed of the devils – was healed'
- Healing remedies – *nathan reph* (Hebrew)
  Ezekiel 30:21 – 'Not be bound up to be healed'
  Jeremiah 46:11 – 'You will use many medicines'

- Natural healing – *kehah* (Hebrew)
  Nahum 3:19 – 'no healing of thy bruise'
- Restoring strength – *tealah* (Hebrew)
  Jeremiah 30:13 – 'you have no healing medicines'

The word *rapha* (Exodus 15:26) also includes gradual healing (to become – Leviticus 13:37), the process of healing (to cause – Exodus 21:19) and the allowing of oneself to be healed i.e. personal responsibility in healing (to allow oneself – 2 Kings 8:29). Healing emphasises repair, restoration and responsibility in the process of healing. It also takes it beyond the personal into how the church can bring healing in the land (2 Chronicles 7:14).

2. Health (divine or biblical)

1. *'Beloved, I pray that you may prosper in all things and be in health, just as your soul prospers.* **3 John 1:2**
2. *'And the very God of peace sanctify you wholly; and I pray God your whole spirit and soul and body be preserved blameless unto the coming of our Lord Jesus Christ'.* **1 Thessalonians 5:23**

Health is more than restoring what is lost or repairing what has been broken; it relates to your functional capacity, dynamic of living (not just existing) and fulfilment of purpose.

'Health is more than restoring what is lost or repairing what has been broken; it relates to your functional capacity, dynamic of living and fulfilment of purpose.'

It has variously been defined as a sense of well being but more than that the health ideal states:

A state of being, bodily and mentally vigorous, free from disease and finding spiritual fulfilment.

An analogy of health:
A car with a flat tyre is repaired and ready to go. However, with no oil in the engine, petrol in the tank, driver behind the wheel or direction in which to drive it is static, functionless and purposeless. Health takes you beyond the state of restoration and repair into purpose, function, potential and possibility.

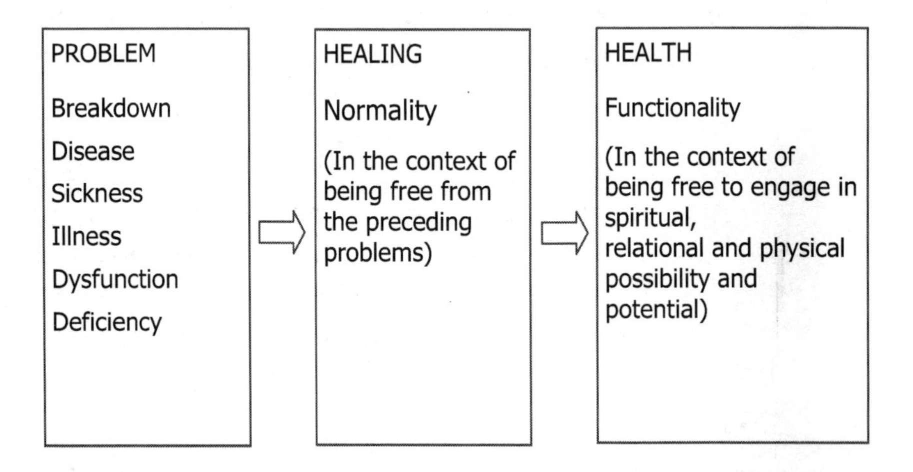

Remember that biblical health is simply being all that God wants you to be – in your marriage, family, friendships, life, ministry, mind and body. It is about being a whole person in a whole community for a whole nation. That is the ideal process of biblical health.

Healing helps make you 'free from'; health empowers you to be 'free to'. As a state of being and not a state of doing, it is not just about what you become – it is about what you are created to be.

3. Life (divine or biblical)
John 10:10

'*The thief cometh not, but for to steal, and to kill, and to destroy: I am come that they might have life, and that they might have it more abundantly'.*

The thief coming is not a maybe or could be – he will come, he has come and he does come with a three-pronged focus; theft, murder and destruction. There is life and there is life more abundantly, which is not automatic. This kind of life has a specific meaning as opposed to being alive (*chai* {Hebrew} – Genesis 2:7); length of days (*yomayim* {Hebrew} – Psalms 91:16); breath (*nephesh* {Hebrew} – Genesis 9:4); physical life (*etsem* {Hebrew} – Job 7:15); life in the world (*biotikos* {Greek} – Luke 21:34); how you've lived (*biosis* {Greek} – Acts 26:4) and the course of your life (*agoge* {Greek} – 2 Timothy 3:10).

The life in John 10:10 is '*Zoë'* (Greek) which relates to the God nature, God-related, God kind of life that is in Christ and in eternity. This takes us beyond mere healing and health to a God quality, eternal quality of God in which we partake in Him. The 'I am' of God defines some of the qualities of this life through which health and healing can come to us but also provides the central point of grace and unconditional love upon which we base our health and healing; His name denotes His nature:

- The Lord our righteousness – Jeremiah 23:6 Jehovah *Tsidkenu* (Hebrew)
- The Lord who sanctifies you – Exodus 31:13 Jehovah *M'kaddesh* (Hebrew)
- The Lord is peace – Judges 6:24 Jehovah *Shalom* (Hebrew)
- The Lord is there – Ezekiel 48:35 Jehovah *Shammah* (Hebrew)
- The Lord who heals – Exodus 15:26 – Jehovah *Rapha* (Hebrew)
- The Lord will provide – Genesis 22:13-14 Jehovah *Jireh* (Hebrew)
- The Lord is my shepherd – Psalms 23:1 Jehovah *Rohi* (Hebrew)
- The Lord is my banner – Exodus 17:15 Jehovah *Nissi* (Hebrew)
- The Lord of hosts – Isaiah 3:1 Jehovah *Sabaoth* (Hebrew)

The word *'Zoe'* life defines a life that is in motion and that has activity. To possess the God kind of life means to be fully alive in Him. It is not merely existing. 'Zoe' life is what He is in us; health is what we become in Him.

Health is the motion towards having and living the God kind of life that will be fulfilled in us in eternity. We have life in Christ but we then live more abundantly. To live abundantly is to be more abundantly alive.

> *'Health is the motion towards having and living the God kind of life that will be fulfilled in us in eternity. We have life in Christ but then we live more abundantly. To live abundantly is to be more abundantly alive.'*

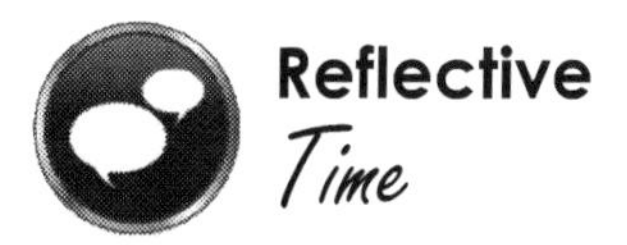

(30 minutes)

1. **What do I have and do to a minimum in my life?**
2. **What do I have and do to maintain my life in its present state?**
3. **What do I have and do to a maximum in my life?**
4. **How can I fulfil more of my potential?**

Personal *Thoughts*

C. PRINCIPLES OF BIBLICAL HEALTH

There are 3 important concepts that clearly distinguish health in the bible from health in the world. Most belief systems have a concept of health (e.g. conventional medicine is based on a Greek model, traditional Chinese medicine on a balance of Yin versus Yang, Ayurvedic medicine is based on some holistic principles of Hinduism). Judeo Christian health, as related in the bible, is distinct and different.

1. Regeneration

This means:

- **To be formed or form again**
- **To come or to bring into existence**
- **To replace with new growth**
- **To cause to replace with new**

Biblical health is not just the capacity to repair what is broken or restore what is lost, it is the power of God to make new or make new again. It is a creative power that was exercised in creation in creative power but in the new creation (2 Corinthians 5:17) in regeneration.

It also operated biblically in turning around situations, making the impossible possible, performing miracles and in doing new things (Isaiah 43:19). Regeneration is unique to God and is uniquely biblical. It is vital in health when the old or damaged is so disrupted as to make restoration or repair impossible.

Regeneration has the power to make new and includes the potential for things to be made new, the process by which things are made new and the replacement of what is no longer working (e.g. the oxygen carrying cells in the body – the red blood cells are completely replaced by new ones; that is natural regeneration).

The only hope for a marriage on the point of divorce is regeneration. When restoration and reconciliation have failed, regeneration can still work.

2. Wholeness

I prefer the word wholeness to holism for two reasons :–

Holistic sometimes generates negative associations for Christians and can be a stumbling block as the word is often associated with New Age. Wholeness extends beyond holistic. Holism is the idea that the whole is greater than the sum of the parts, that there is a synergistic or additive effect. For example, when you add together yeast, flour, water and salt they are the constituents of bread. But when mixed and heated the yeast causes the bread to rise. The product is a loaf of bread as a result of the mixing and heating. Holism is that process.

As humans we are integrated entities. Our spirit interrelates with our soul, which in turn relates with our body (e.g. a broken marriage can lead to a spiritually wounded minister and a physical stress ulcer). Wholeness, however, takes it a step further and says that each part has a capacity of its own and in order for the total person to be whole each part must be functioning effectively and integrating correctly with the rest. This is the essence of biblical health. It is a concept of being complete or having completeness. It is a dynamic relationship where the relationship between each part is as important as each part (e.g. if a person has a tremendous insight into the spiritual nature of marriage but is not able to translate that to practical daily life with his spouse, the relationship between spirit and soul is dysfunctional). Equally a vibrant ministry that neglects the physical well being of the body will eventually be hampered in its capacity due to resultant illness or physical restrictions.

'Wholeness says that each part has a capacity of its own. In order for the total person to be whole each part must be functioning correctly. This is the essence of biblical health.'

3. Characteristics of the human personality

The biblical basis for a human being is a triune personality consisting of distinct but interrelated, interdependent parts making up the whole. These parts are the spirit, soul and the body of a person. To define a human on earth, all three must be present. To define total health all three must be functioning as God intended in relation to him, to each other and to the world around it.

1. Spirit

This is the central part of the triune personality. It is the seat of devotion, worship, love and peace amongst other things. It is the place of deepest desire and fulfilment. This can only be truly fulfilled through a genuine living relationship with God through Jesus Christ in unconditional love and grace.

2. Soul

This is the relational part of the personality. It is the interactional pivotal point through which many issues of relationship pass including the mind (intellect, memory and imagination), emotions and choice. Much of the transfer and communication comes via our senses.

3. Body

This has a temporal state and it is a vehicle of containment and function.
It links with the spirit in being the physical temple of the Holy Spirit and the person's own spirit. It links with the soul through the senses.

These three are not just integrated and distinct parts of our person but have definitive God given order of priority in importance and operation. God is a spirit (John 4:24) and our spiritual identity defines who we are at the most fundamental level (see later).

God created the world and all that is in it for relationship at some level. Our soul is affected by our deepest spiritual state and drives our physical life in response to its condition (e.g. sexual abuse in childhood can often lead to

abusive relationships later in life). Our physical bodies help facilitate our spiritual and soulish state to achieve their purpose (1 Timothy 4:8; 1 Corinthians 6:19-20). A healthy body can lead to a healthier mind.
All three distinct entities are important but God's creative order is:

1st – Spirit

2nd – Soul

3rd – Body

As we will see later, the fallen world operates in exact reverse and hence we see many of the results in our societies today.

Reflective *Time*

(30 minutes)

1. **What areas of my life need regeneration?**
2. **In what area do I find it difficult to translate my spiritual experience into practical daily reality?**
3. **In what areas is my life not spirit, soul and body?**
4. **What can I do to change my priorities?**

Personal *Thoughts*

D. JESUS THE MAN OF HEALTH

1. His ministry

It is noteworthy that from the beginning of Jesus' ministry He engaged in healing and ministry involving the whole person.

'The Spirit of the Lord is upon Me, because He has anointed Me to preach the gospel to the poor, He has sent Me to heal the broken-hearted, to proclaim liberty to the captives, and recovery of sight to the blind, to set at liberty those who are oppressed; To proclaim the acceptable year of the Lord.'
Luke 4:18-19

The Holy Spirit's anointing, from descending upon Him (Luke 3:22), filling, leading (Luke 4:1) and empowering Him (Luke 4:14), brought Him to the place of Luke 4:18 where God clearly had a spirit, soul and body agenda. Many of the specifics in Luke 4:18 can be applied to many aspects of the human personality but some distinctions include:

Preaching the gospel – spirit
Preaching deliverance – spirit/soul
Healing the broken hearted – spirit/soul
Sight to the blind – spirit/soul/body
Liberty to the bruised – spirit/soul
Acceptable year – spirit/soul/body

Many of the gospel accounts of healing and miracles involved much more than the physical effect and response. Jesus often saw beyond the need presented to Him to respond to the real need of the person. A beautiful example of this is the story of the woman with the issue of blood in Mark 5:21-34. Several points to note from this story:

- **She had prolonged menstrual bleeding**
- **She had it for 12 years**

- **She was bankrupt**
- **She was unclean and as such rejected**
- **She was desperate**

Her desperation showed in several things:

- **She was in the locality when she would be expected to be indoors with her bleeding problem**
- **She was willing to touch a religious man (not generally acceptable as an unclean person)**
- **She was willing to touch the Raboni – chief Rabbi of Rabbis, most religious of religious in the eyes of people – Jesus**

Jesus then called out 'who touched me?' and made her situation apparently even worse by making it public in front of the whole crowd. His response then summarised total healing of spirit, soul and body:

1. **He called her daughter. Her faith brought her into spiritual relationship with the Father**
2. **She was made whole and restored in relationship as He told her to 'go in peace'**
3. **Her physical plague was healed**

'Many of the gospel accounts of healing and miracles involved much more than the physical effect and response. Jesus often saw beyond the need presented to the real need of the person.'

2. His Life

Jesus exhibited total health within Himself. He lived a short life but exhibited a strong relationship with His Father, epitomised in Luke 3:21-22 and John chapters 14 and 17. He understood correct alignment in relationship to His parents (Luke 2:51), to the local church (Luke 4:16), to leadership (Luke 2:46) and to the law of the land (Matthew 2:21). He experienced community (Luke 4:16 and 22), friendship (John 15:15), fellowship (John 12:1-2) and emotions (John 11:3). He had a broad circle of relationships with people of varied backgrounds and education. He was teachable and increased in knowledge and learning from an early age (Luke 1:80; 2:52). There was no record of sickness in His life and He fulfilled His purpose in life (Luke 9:51-56).

It is recorded that His life was so full of words and deeds that if books were written the world could not contain all that was said about Him (John 21:25). He had a remarkable life and died at 33 years old and yet even in His death on the cross there is a pointer to total health for us. It is through the cross that spiritual health can be restored, interpersonal health finds hope and physical health finds healing. We cannot attain all that Jesus did as sickness has already plagued every one of our bodies at some point in our lifetime. We can however take heart, have hope and put faith upon what He did for us on the cross.

3. His Death

In the account of what Jesus took upon Himself on the cross in Isaiah 53:4-12 and I Peter 2:24 we see a clear reference to many levels and areas of suffering. I will go into more detail with this later but I want to summarise certain areas:

- **Spiritual**
  Iniquity – Isaiah 53:5-10; 1 Peter 2:4-24
- **Soulish**
  Grief, sorrows – Isaiah 53:4
- **Physical**
  Stripes – Isaiah 53:5; 1 Peter 2:24

In His life, ministry and death Jesus epitomised biblical health in its entirety. He is our example and role model. He was a true man of health who fully practised all He preached. There is no man in history who has carried divine healing, divine health and divine life in such total measure as Jesus Christ.

'There is no man in history who has carried divine healing, divine health and divine life in such total measure as Jesus Christ.'

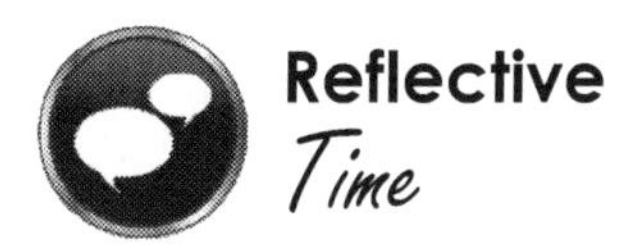

(20 minutes)

Read the Gospels and answer the following questions:

1. **Identify times and incidents where Jesus ministered in a whole person way**
2. **Identify times and incidents in Jesus' life that demonstrate that He lived in a whole person way**
3. **Reflect upon reasons why Jesus ministered to the whole person as in the example of the woman with the issue of blood**

Personal *Thoughts*

....

....

....

....

....

....

....

....

....

....

SECTION TWO - HEALTH OF THE SPIRIT

CHAPTER TWO

PURPOSE

Faith and spirituality is a huge topic and I have restricted the material in this section to that which relates more directly to health issues.

Introduction

'To find your purpose in life'. This was included in one of the definitions of health we looked at earlier. Lack of purpose can reveal itself in many ways; lack of direction, motivation, emptiness, incompleteness, drifting, waywardness, indecision and even elements of mental illness and suicide. Society has changed over the past 100 years. We no longer live in a 'man's world'. This has many positive aspects but men can feel a lack of importance in their role as husbands, fathers, workers and societal members.

Women's role in society has changed tremendously. Their health profile has changed due to long working hours in addition to home life, stress and increased amounts of alcohol and smoking. They are now suffering from the traditional male diseases of lung cancer and heart disease.

Purpose is a fundamental part of health. It is an issue which is rarely addressed and is like an iceberg in people's lives. People rarely talk about their need to have purpose in life but everyone is seeking purpose and significance in life.

At times of crises people look at these more fundamental issues and realise that there is a lot 'lying beneath the surface' of their lives that has never been properly addressed. Purpose is about finding your place, function and significance in life and relationships.

'Purpose is a fundamental part of health. It is finding your place, function and significance in life and relationships.'

'My meat is to do the will of Him that sent me and to finish His work'.
John 4:34

These were Jesus' words when challenged by physical need for food. He was clearly on a journey and had a purpose to fulfil.
Purpose is an outworking of three other principle questions:

1. Who am I?
2. Where am I?
3. What am I?

1. Who am I?

This deals with fundamental identity as human beings. It is a question that is rarely asked but always necessary. As one person said – 'There is a God-shaped hole in all of us that can only be filled by Him'.

One medical journal asked in June 2003 'Is God in the Yellow Pages?' Where can I find Him? Philosophy states that you can't have something from nothing. The missing link is creation or in the words of a U.S. astronomer 'To make an apple pie from scratch you must first create the universe'. I think that puts it in perspective.

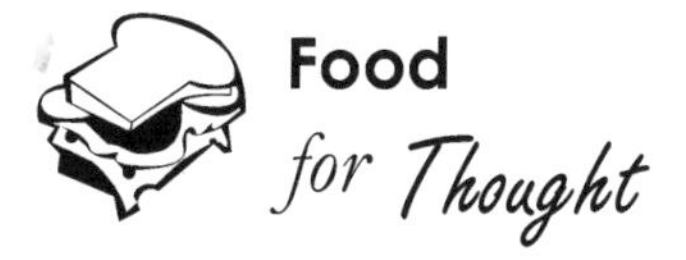

A nurse once asked Albert Einstein 'Is there an answer to everything? He replied 'I think that to everything there is an answer'. The world is too busy asking the question to think about the answer

What is the central point around which the fundamental questions of life are answered? Creation demands a creator, a creator poses a possibility of relationship and a relationship projects upon identity.

Religion has a form of God; the bible makes a friend of God. Fundamental spiritual identity is based upon trust in God as your Father through faith in His Son Jesus Christ.

This is a blood covenant of unconditional nature in love and grace. If our identity rests upon anything else it will falter. If the devil can destroy your identity he can undermine your destiny.

2. Where am I?

This deals with our security in time, place and person. Security within us is the fundamental sense of how we think, feel, believe and know. This is not governed by the negative or dysfunctional expectations, demands and influences of our relational environment. It is founded in our identity.
If God took our ministry away from us tomorrow, would we love Him the same, live for Him the same and serve Him the same? A security that is based upon a wrong identity is always dysfunctional and often dangerous. Sonship (and daughtership) is unmerited adoption that is legally and totally binding. We are the sons and daughters that serve and not servants trying to become sons. One is rooted in grace and the other in law. Parenting, marriage, ministry and leadership must be founded on a secure identity in Christ and a level of personal wholeness.

- **Security in time**

This deals with the relationship of our identity to our past, present and future. To our past in dealing with parenting, genetics, education, peers, relationships (e.g. soul ties, abuse, neglect, fear, rejection and favouritism can be factors affecting our security within ourselves as individuals). To the present in relation to where we are today (are we the same in the pulpit as in the pew, public as in private, personal as in relational?). The future relates to ambitions, deadlines, goals and fear of failure. Authentic life is secure in time.

- **Security in place**

This deals with the relationship of our identity to where we are at in our lives today. This may have a material focus i.e. possessions, a disability or limitation, or a feeling of educational disadvantage. These can generate unrealistic or wrong expectations and demands. It can breed an unfair and ungodly dissatisfaction and discontentment that can reinforce low self-esteem.

Some people are always discontent because they have a materialistic focus or an unrealistic ambition that is based on their desires rather than God's will. Some people cannot find rest in situations of conflict because of guilt or they feel they should have the answers. Secure people find rest in God's will.

- **Security in person**

This deals with the relationship of your identity with the real you of your past. As a faith issue, identity and security in Christ takes you outside of yourself and into Him. There is always this 'Egypt syndrome' of tending to look back and feel secure in the comfort of our past, even if it is dysfunctional. This is symbolic of the children of Israel in the wilderness in the Old Testament.

Guilt and past failure want to sabotage that simple faith in a loving father. A childlike trust in the goodness of God is necessary to keep us in love, in grace, in peace and in the security of knowing that nothing can separate us from the love of God (Romans 8:35-39).
In this we can find rest within ourselves despite our past or present circumstances and experiences.

- **Your identity defines who you really are**
- **Your security defines where you are really at**
- **Both are necessary to find real purpose**

3. What am I?

This defines your role and your function. A dysfunctional identity and security that is tied irreversibly to role or function can be a dangerous cocktail. We can then become position or title orientated and can lose ourselves in the role, become self-willed and lose accountability and humility. Each role we play as spouses, ministers, civilians, children, and society members has potential for defining our identity or security in totality. The essence of biblical health lies in the ability to hold all the different areas of our lives in correct role and responsibility but in a spirit, soul, and body order.

Our identity and security in Christ is worked out in a passionate, grateful devotional life that becomes evident in our relationship to our spouse and family before being demonstrated in life, ministry, physical discipline and development. This then becomes the bedrock for identifying and fulfilling God-given purpose in life.

4. Why am I?

Purpose defines why am I? This question encompasses aspects of the preceding three but can also follow on from that. Purpose means the reason for which something is done.

There are several aspects to purpose:

- **Creative Purpose - Revelation 4:11**

'We are created for His pleasure'.

This purpose is fulfilled in answering who am I affirmatively (i.e. being secure in your identity) and living that out effectively. If we please God through faith and trust in Him we can be fulfilled in our creative purpose.

- **Relational Purpose - Genesis 2:18**

'It is not good that the man should be alone...'

This purpose is only fulfilled through relationships. Single parent mums have a higher rate of suicide, depression and accidents than married ones. There is a need in all of us for close personal, trusting relationships. Wholeness in this area is necessary to answer 'where am I' positively.

- **Universal Purpose - Genesis 1:27-28**

'So God created man in His own image, in the image of God He created him, male and female He created them. Then God blessed them, and God said to them "Be fruitful and multiply; fill the earth and subdue it; have dominion...".'

Rights and responsibilities, authority and accountability, influence and integrity are the two faces of one coin that we all carry in the wallet of this world. There is great blessing in this promise but it comes with a huge responsibility that we all share. Procreation and prosperity are commandments that find their purpose and meaning in the gospel. Sexual relations outside of marriage, alternative styles of family life, and man's quest for comfort and global power struggles all demonstrate the daily challenges in the world to God's perfect creative design.

- **Ministry Purpose – Romans 12:3**

'According as God hath dealt to every man the measure of faith.'

There is a measure of faith to exercise gifts according to the grace given and what the limits are for us. William Shakespeare said 'Some are born great, some achieve greatness and some have greatness thrust upon them'. Ordinary people can do extraordinary things in the purposes of God. Let God set your limits based on His expectations for you. We tend to see our cup half empty; God tends to see it half full. It is not what you lack; it is what He has that determines outcome. Utilising our God-given gifts, talents and time activates purpose and provides fulfilment in our lives.

- **Personal Purpose – John 15:16**

'You have not chosen me, but I have chosen you, and ordained you, that you should go and bring forth fruit, and that your fruit should remain.'

Your personal purpose is God's unique and specific task, direction, training and reason for your life. All the preceding purposes are important and relevant but this is your personal journey with God that can include a 'specific' calling to a certain area of life and ministry. There are numerous examples of this in the bible and even in the lives of great men and women of history. The following are common threads that run in a personal purpose:

1. An origin - An encounter with God, a personal conflict or struggle, a sense of destiny
2. A vision - 'Many see but they have no vision' said a great artist. Vision sees you and then you see it. Visionaries look at the same thing, but see something different. When Jesus called Peter into the ministry He called him Peter the rock, everyone else saw Simon the reed. Purpose requires a sense of direction and direction requires a sense of vision
3. A process - 2007 is the 200th anniversary of the abolition of the slave trade in the UK. William Wilberforce was on his deathbed when it finally happened. He had been battling most of his political life for the abolition of the slave trade and reformation of society. Jim Elliot wrote in his journal hours before being martyred in South America 'He is no fool who gives what he cannot keep to gain what he cannot lose'. Purpose links us to the generation before us, the generation we are living in and the generation after us. It is God's thread through the ages that weaves His eternal plan. Our lifetime is but one stitch but it is His 'stitch in time' that reflects our lives. Purpose is a process and not just the product. You have one lifetime to be an active part of the process
4. A promise - Total spiritual health is to find and fulfil all the purposes I have mentioned above. It begins in Christ, becomes for Christ and ends with Christ. Our personal purpose is a necessary part of the whole and sadly many live safe to stay in the middle of the road. God is a risk taker and not a risk manager. Bertrand Russel said 'The most insecure people on earth

are those who are forever playing it safe'. You can have the greatest marriage, the greatest physical health, and the largest house, but if you are not finding and fulfilling your purpose in life you are not in health. Purpose is a journey with a specific sense of completion or accomplishment. There is a promise over our lives of the potential within us. If we realise this potential then we have fulfilled the promise

Summary

Spiritual health answers all four questions clearly.

Who am I?

Where am I?

What am I

Why am I?

These questions deal with your identity and security as a person, your role in life, society and ministry and your reasons for living. Issues of spiritual health are often neglected when addressing general wellbeing and health. They are however pivotal points of unhappiness, breakdown, and emptiness in people's lives that undermine all other aspects of health.

Issues of spiritual health are fundamental to the authentic voice of the church today. They are points of contact between society and the gospel. A lack of purpose can create a feeling of emptiness, unfulfilment and regret. Jesus was a man of purpose who said on the cross 'It is finished' (John 19:30). He had fulfilled the purpose for which He was born which was primarily spiritual to redeem mankind back to a loving Father. May we be able to end our lives uttering the same words?

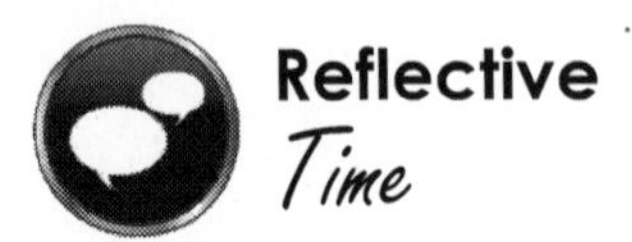

(20 minutes)

1. **What unresolved issues are there in your identity and security?**
2. **Do you have accountability in all areas of your life - ministry, marriage, finance, personal and private?**
3. **Are you fulfilled in all areas of purpose, and if not, why?**

Personal *Thoughts*

SECTION THREE - HEALTH OF THE SOUL

CHAPTER THREE

THE MIND: BATTLEGROUND, PLAYGROUND OR GROUND-BREAKING

1. Introduction

For many people, their mental horizon is what they've known, seen, understood and reasoned. The world was flat to most except Christopher Columbus. It made perfect sense at the time but Christopher Columbus trusted God and set sail to test the hypothesis. He found that his hypothesis was correct and the earth was not flat. Many people have never tested the hypothesis of what their mind is capable of in God.

Before I address that, I want to look at the mental state of the nation. Mental health, particularly among the young, is a worrying trend. Suicide rates have increased in young men in recent years. Binge drinking and recreational drugs have consequences upon psychological state. The vast majority of crimes are still drug and alcohol related. Depression is the second most common disability next to heart disease in the UK and it is estimated that 1 in 4 people in the UK have a mental health problem. Antisocial behaviour and gang warfare is a part of inner city (and many rural communities) life.
With societies redefining the family, marriage and values, we are reaping the whirlwind in this generation. 80-90 per cent of children in juvenile crime come from broken homes and families. 40 per cent of babies are born outside of marriage with 28 per cent to single parents; 98 per cent of single parents are women. This is creating a fatherless generation of frightening proportions.

Memories, imaginations and thoughts are tainted by experiences of childhood, parenting, peers and society as a whole. Hardness of heart, lack of natural empathy and heartlessness seem rampant in this fractured and fragmented society in which we live. Before we can function in capacity we need to address incapacity.

Mental ill health has many sources and many solutions to help recovery but I will focus on the transformation of the mind into mental capacity to move from illness to healing to health.

There are 2 issues to address here:

- **Mental Capacity**
- **Mental Incapacity**

2. Mental Incapacity

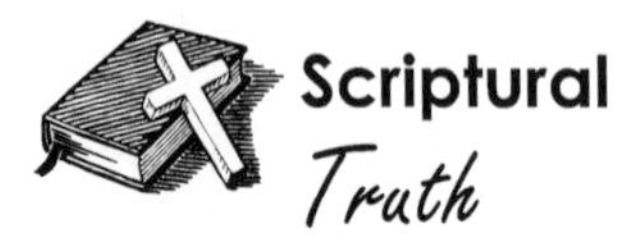

'For the weapons of our warfare are not carnal, but mighty through God to the pulling down of strongholds; Casting down imaginations, and every high thing that exalteth itself against the knowledge of God, and bringing into captivity every thought to the obedience of Christ.' **2 Corinthians 10:4-5**

A stronghold is a fortress with walls. Its aim is to confine you within a certain frame of thinking. People with depression frame everything within the reference of their low mood. Some people are held by their cultural or racial limits, some by their family expectations. The transformation of the mind is to bring every thought to the obedience of Christ. Evan Roberts, a pioneer in the 1904 Welsh Revival of Christianity received four keys from God to revival:

1. **Confess sin**
2. **Deal with doubtful areas**
3. **Immediate obedience to the Holy Spirit**
4. **Confess Christ publicly.**

The above principles can help us to live in mental health and not breakdown. Many people live with internal conflicts that destroy their soul and spirit.

Renewed thinking

Believe the witness and obey the prompting of the Holy Spirit however contrary to your frame of reference (e.g. some women who have experienced sexual abuse find it difficult to experience intimacy in a further relationship). The scripture, *'I am fearfully and wonderfully made...that my soul knoweth right well'* (Psalm 139:14) needs to be a personal witness to break free from the stronghold of abuse and bad experience.

- **Deal with disappointments**

'A man should never be ashamed to own he has been wrong, which is but saying, that he is wiser today than he was yesterday' - Alexander Pope (1688 – 1744). Most great leaders become such not because they know how to deal with success but because they learned how to deal with failure.

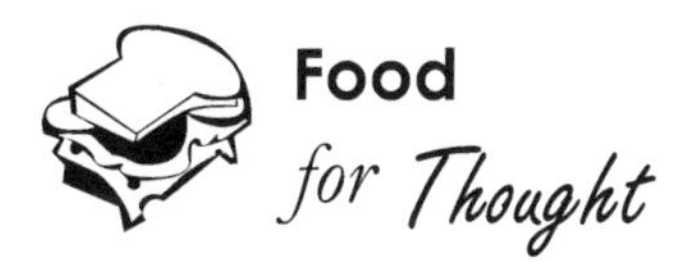

'When I look back on all these worries I remember the story of the old man who said on his deathbed that he had had a lot of trouble in his life, most of which had never happened' – Winston Churchill

- **Don't believe a lie - worry**

You will never know what you can do until you do it. You can never know what you can be until you become it.

- **Develop your mind**

Adam named all the animals. This took tremendous capacity and potential. 'Discoveries are often made by going off the main road and by trying the untried' – Frank Tyer.

- **Keep learning new things**

On studying longevity of life one of the characteristics that were common to them was not just faith and marriage, but the presence of a pioneering spirit defined as an interest in new things and an enthusiasm for change.

- **Study**

'*Study to shew thyself approved unto God, a workman that needeth not to be ashamed, rightly dividing the word of truth'.* **2 Timothy 2:15**

- **Don't fear change**

'*And be not conformed to this world: but be ye transformed by the renewing of your mind, that ye may prove what is that good, and acceptable, and perfect, will of God'.* **Romans 12:2**

- Conforming means no change (other than to what's around you)
- Transforming means to change
- Renewal means to change again

'By nature man hates change, seldom will he quit his old home till it has actually fallen around his ears' - Thomas Carlyle (1795-1881).

The six D's of change are:

Deliberate	– decide what you want to change
Dream	– consider all possibilities
Describe	– be precise about what you want to do
Discuss	– talk to relevant people
Decide	– on the steps you will take to achieve
Do it	– take action

3. Mental Capacity

The mind is a powerful entity. God created it to be a vehicle of thought, imagination, memory and creativity.

- Adam named the animals (Genesis 2:19-20)
- Jesus remembered the word 'it is written' (Luke 4:4,8,12)
- Solomon spoke 3000 proverbs and 1005 songs (1 Kings 4:32)
- Daniel was skilful in wisdom, gifted in knowledge, and understood science, visions and dreams (Daniel 1:4-17)

We have the mind of Christ, which enlightens and empowers our natural mind to think outside the box. A mind that is mindless will wander and a brain that is static will probably gravitate to negativity.

'Finally my brothers, whatever things are true, whatever things are honest, whatever things are just, whatever things are pure, whatever things are lovely, whatever things are of a good report, if there be any virtue and if there be any praise, think on these things. And the peace of God, which passes all understanding, shall keep your hearts and minds in Christ Jesus.'
Philippians 4:7-8

Final Thought:

A definition of mental health was proposed which encapsulates exactly the characteristics of a biblical health model:

'The emotional and spiritual resilience which enables us to enjoy life, to survive disappointment and sadness. It is a positive sense of well-being and an underlying belief in our own and others dignity and worth'.

This not only includes responding to mental incapacity but also embracing mental capacity. **Most people are content with not living in a state of mental incapacity. God has more for you than that. He wants you to fulfil your potential.**

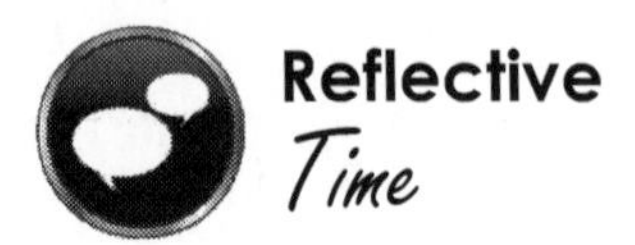

(20 minutes)

1. **Are there persistent, intrusive thoughts that you struggle with?**
2. **What limitations do you place on your thinking?**
3. **How would you develop your mind further in God?**

If you are troubled by persistent thoughts that affect your mental state, you should consult a medical doctor

Personal *Thoughts*

CHAPTER FOUR

EMOTIONS: PAST, PRESENT OR FUTURE

Introduction

Deep-seated emotions such as fear, shame, and rejection can be destructive and debilitating. Feelings are present to give us a sense of emotion and expression. They are a vehicle through which spiritual love, joy, peace and passion can be channelled.

The biblical word 'heart' can be associated with emotions as well as the spiritual nature of a person. It relates to the 'bowel' or 'inside of a person', the 'centre' and being in the 'midst'.

Isaiah 53

This chapter highlights some of the very deep-seated emotions associated with Jesus' life and death:

Verse 2 – no form or comeliness – *image, looks and appearance.*

I am not a person obsessed with image but I do understand from personal experience what it means to have a distorted body image - anorexia, bulimia and more subtle things of discontentment with yourself physically. We can be forever comparing, competing or contrasting.

An advertising campaign for Nike made the statement 'image is everything'. How true, but it depends upon which image you believe of yourself. Negative self-image can dominate the whole focus of your life. 'We are created in God's image and likeness' (Genesis 1:26). Some people's fear and shame is rooted in image. Image is what you reflect upon yourself, upon others and upon life.

What you reflect is what you resemble and what you resemble is what you represent. If you reflect rejection, because that is the image you have within yourself, you will resemble rejection in how you relate, how you feel and what you believe about yourself and others and you will represent rejection by the following - you will reject and you will be rejected because like attracts like. If you find acceptance in God then your outlook will be more whole.

Verse 2 — no beauty that we should desire

Most women secretly wish in their unregenerate days that every man would turn their head to look at them and most men would wish that women were whispering with sparkling eyes when they walk past. But Jesus had no beauty that would cause desire. Maybe you wish that you were desired. Maybe you think there is something wrong with you because you are not desired. Single people may struggle with this. What's wrong with me? Crisis of confidence. Some leaders gauge their self-esteem by the Sunday turnout.

Verse 3 — despised, rejected

These are strong words. These things impinge upon our soul and wound our spirit.

Verse 3 — a man of sorrows and acquainted with grief.

This indicates being familiar with, or understanding grief (a deep sense of sadness as a result of loss). Grief can be tied to abandonment and separation. The level of grief is not determined by the level of loss but by the reflection of that loss upon a person's life. Some people can lose some major things and be moderately affected by grief. Others can suffer minor loss but be severely traumatised.

As a medical doctor I often examine patients after a car accident for their medico legal claim. It never ceases to amaze me now how little you can predict a person's response to an accident. You can have someone whose car was flipped over and thrust to the other side of the road and they get up unscathed - no nightmares, no tears, little problem with getting into a car again. You can have someone else with a slight bump at a red light and they have post traumatic stress disorder. Grief is a deep sadness that clouds a person's spirit. You may have lost your cat or a spouse of 50 years. It is how the bereavement is reflected upon you that determines the level of grief and your response.

Verse 3 – hid our faces from Him

Shame is an uncomfortable self-consciousness that causes a person to recoil, withdraw, or hide. It is a self-effacement, making you inconspicuous and wanting to withdraw. It can inhibit people emotionally and physically, like a rabbit in the road when the light shines. The rabbit feels uncovered and exposed and it becomes momentarily 'paralysed.'

Verse 5 – He was wounded

A breakage of a barrier – the skin – an open wound. When the protective barrier is violated or crossed over. Wounds leave scar tissue. It's the mark or the evidence that a wound has taken place. A wound occurs when someone is violated, transgressed (breaking of an agreement or covenant) or a boundary crossed, as in abuse. It leaves people feeling sensitive and exposed.

Verse 5 – bruised

That is hidden bleeding. Haemorrhage that is evident but not visible. They are haemorrhaging inside but you don't see the blood; you see the effect of the blood in the bruise. Like a child who has been told off, you can ask them if they are all right – they say yes but often they mean no. They are angry, frustrated and disappointed inside. This is evident in their tone, body language or demeanour. People may recognise the bruise and that something is not right in their lives but they don't know the source. Jesus knows the real issues.

We tend to focus on Isaiah 53 verse 5 which states that 'by His stripes we are healed'. We often focus on the physical associated with the verse and that is important but most of what Isaiah wrote in chapter 53 in relation to Jesus' death was the emotional, the psychological and the spiritual.

'The spirit of a man will sustain his infirmity; but a wounded spirit who can bear?' **Proverbs 18:14**

In the recent Hollywood movie 'Rocky Balboa' starring Sylvester Stallone there is a wonderful statement towards the end of the film. It says 'The last thing to age is your heart'. In the area of emotional healing I want to encourage you to 'give your heart a chance'. Allow God to heal and restore it and let it be free to express passion, worship, love and commitment.

How can we find emotional healing?

1. Choice

The soul is hinged on the will. You have to determine to want to change and be determined to change.

There is no growth without change and there is no change without conflict and there is no conflict without tension. You have to choose to change. No choice – no change. You shall know the truth and the truth shall MAKE you free **(John 8:31-32)**

Know the truth – you are not what you were. The woman with the issue of blood (Mark 5:24-34). Her issue was not just the blood; it was rejection, image and self-esteem. She touched Him. Blind Bartimaeus cried out 'Jesus' - until he got Jesus' attention (Mark 10:46-52). Jesus asked Bartimaeus 'What do you want me to do for you?'

For some, healing comes through a godly relationship, for others the laying on of hands or perhaps counselling, but for all it's an act of faith in decision. You have to make a home in the truth however unfamiliar and uncomfortable that is to your experience.

2. Chosen

Luke 4:21 – 'Today' Jesus said – this scripture is fulfilled in your ears. Scripture is fulfilled. To be full and filled with the scripture. Some people really underestimate the power of the written truth of scripture. They relate to modern day and try and interpret doctrine in relation to modern trends and beliefs. Scripture stands alone however as the very essence of truth. It is complete within itself. In this area of emotions we are so programmed and patterned and formed by our upbringing, environment, fallen state, dysfunctions and weaknesses that it seems like a permanent bent in our soul. The scripture however must be the absolute literal and final truth upon which we base our belief system. Sometimes people say – 'God said this to me' and in the next breath they contradict by their word or action exactly what they have just claimed to believe.

Some relevant scriptural examples are:

- ***'I AM fearfully and wonderfully made.'* (Psalm 139:14)**

  It isn't enough just to say Amen! Do you understand it? Is it personal truth to you?

- ***'Before I formed YOU in the womb I knew YOU.'* (Jeremiah 1:5)**

  Your parents may not want you but God knew and God does want you.

- ***'Behold I give unto YOU power... and over ALL the power of the enemy.'* (Luke 10:19)**

It is important to understand the grace we are under and the authority we have as children of God.

- ***'Having DONE all, to stand.'* (Ephesians 6:13)**

When you have done all that you know to do then stand on the truth and freedom that Jesus has for you (Galatians 5:1).

Be not conformed but transformed. Conform is to change you to reflect your environment, reform is to change you to change your environment and transform is to change your environment to reflect you.

3 stages of change:

- **Most conform**
- **Some reform**
- **Few transform**

Change you to change your environment and then change your environment to reflect the new you. The devil is mean, cruel and vicious. You have to be ruthless in these principles of freedom.

- **Believe what is right**
- **Speak what is true**
- **Live what is real**

We make choices in life but our great hope emotionally is that God has chosen us to have relationship with Him. A restoration of relationship with God gives us the tools to see restoration within ourselves. Know that you are chosen IN God, FOR God and BY God.

3. Calling

'The Spirit of the Lord IS upon me because He HAS anointed me' (Luke 4:18). *'But as the same anointing teaches you concerning all things, and is true, and is not a lie, and just as it has taught you, you will abide in Him (live, dwell, remain) in Him.'* (1 John 2: 27-28)

The anointment of the Spirit is the spark that lights the candle. It's the touch, it's the change factor, and it's the moment of God that brings the change.

The woman with the issue touched the border of His garment and immediately virtue left Him and her issue ceased. That is the anointment. But the anointing also (the teaching, the guiding, the moulding, the yielding) abides within, it remains, abides and stays – whether you are over the dinner table, in the office or on the tube. It is present when you are assailed with thoughts, bombarded with emotions and surrounded by fears.

It is able to rule your spirit as you give it Lordship in your heart. It can rule and reign and that is what brings daily, lasting, progressive change day by day, week by week, year-by-year transformation into His likeness. We are created in His image, after His likeness. Creation gives us the image of Christ. Following after gives us the likeness of Christ. The anointing is constantly present to heal and to give hope.

Emotional Healing:

- **It's a matter of choice**
- **It's a matter of being chosen**
- **It's a matter of calling**

To see healing requires right choices in life. Its security is in knowing that God was the initiator in the relationship and therefore it is His grace. We do also need the touch of God deep in our soul (anointment) and to know that God's anointing dwells within us, which has His capacity to change us and keep us.

'To see healing requires right choices in life. Its security is in knowing that God was the initiator in the relationship and therefore it is His grace .'

A Renewed Heart

- **Past, present and future**

Once you've dealt with the past, live in the present and look to the future. Don't sit in your present. That's the difference between health and healing. Healing helps deal with your past to bring you to a positive present but health then takes you into your future.

- **Develop new relationships**

If you only relate to what you know, then you will only become what you were and stay where you are. You conform to your counsel and it's important to surround yourself with godly counsel. Psalm 1 expresses this beautifully. Don't stand with the sinners, sit with the scornful or walk with the wicked. Put yourself around people who are carrying the life of God and are growing.

- **Guard your heart**

'Keep thy heart with all diligence for out of it are the issues of life.'
Proverbs 4:23

What goes around comes around. If there has been a weakness, a falling or you have been a victim in a certain area of life, the enemy would want to exploit that when you're at a point of weakness in the future. Recognise your danger points, weaknesses and vulnerable areas and ruthlessly guard them. Apply wisdom and surround yourself with faith and accountability.

- **Learn your love language**

The excellent book by Gary Chapman entitled 'The Five Love Languages' explains wonderfully the aspects of communication that are critical for giving and receiving love.

What makes you feel loved?

- **Words of affirmation**
- **Gifts**

- **Acts of service**
- **Quality time**
- **Physical touch**

When you are able to express love in the language that the other person receives love then you are more likely to be received, understood and experience closeness. Men and women often have a different love language i.e. what makes you feel loved? Individuals in a relationship can have very different needs, expectations and ways in which they give and receive love.
It is important that you recognise your own 'language of communication' and what other people's languages are. Often we will be influenced by our upbringing in these areas. If our parents never demonstrated love through the physical touch of holding hands and hugs then we may find it hard to receive love in this way.

Many marriages break down because people are communicating two different languages in the home. They both love each other and have love for each other but they are not 'being' loved. The word beloved means 'be'loved. It is an active word, not a statement.

'When all the people were baptized, it came to pass that Jesus also was baptized; and while He prayed, the heaven was opened. And the Holy Spirit descended in bodily form like a dove upon Him, and a voice came from heaven which said, "You are My beloved Son; in You I am well pleased".'
Luke 3:21-22

Luke 3:21-22 gives an example of how the Father communicated love to Jesus through gifts (the Holy Spirit), words of affirmation (you are My BELOVED Son), physical touch (the dove sat upon Him), quality time (Jesus prayed and the Father spoke) and acts of service (Jesus was baptised from His obedience).

Identifying your love languages and of those around you can literally change your life, marriage, working relationships and ministry. Fundamental to each person's identity is the desire to be loved. God is love (I John 4:8). Many of us find it hard to see God as He really is i.e. a loving father and receive from God as He desires to give i.e. unconditionally. God desires to communicates to us in a language that we can understand so that we can personally experience His love.

Conclusion

Emotional wholeness is fundamental to healthy relationships. Love is the central point of our emotions and understanding love languages helps to unlock the door to connecting and communicating with God, ourselves and others.

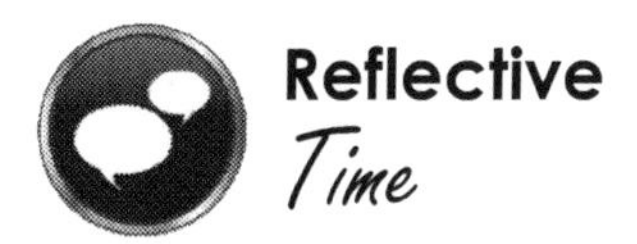

Reflective *Time*

(20 minutes)

1. **What are your unresolved emotional issues?**
2. **What are you doing to guard your heart?**
3. **Name your 2 main love languages and give an example of each and how they have affected you and your life?**
4. **How can you improve your relationships?**

Personal *Thoughts*

CHAPTER FIVE

THE WILL: TO DO OR NOT TO DO

Free will is the most precious and yet risky thing that God gave to man. The potential for destiny and the potential for disaster are both huge possibilities. Decisions determine destiny and sometimes destination.

'See, I have set before thee this day life and good, death and evil.'
Deuteronomy 30:15

Fundamental to faith is the act of obedience. Biblically we serve a king and live in a kingdom. Democracy is a political process not a biblical process, though some of its principles of equity and fairness may be biblical. Modern society has rebelled against authority and its commandments. Consequently, many people struggle with the absolutes of God and the requirement for obedience. The fear of the Lord is a necessary ingredient in responding positively. When we only yield to our own will then we operate in our strength. When we yield to His will we operate in His strength.

A Renewed Will

- **He chose us – We chose Him**

John 15:16

He has already chosen you. We need to die daily to our self will. Choose Him every day. A yielded spirit is not a broken spirit. God allows us freedom of choice. Brokenness produces yieldedness and is the product of the realisation that you can't do it yourself and you need God. You can then yield to God. Yieldedness without brokenness is only psychology and has no power. A broken spirit has lost its desire to choose. It's a type of a wounded spirit that results from trauma. Brokenness without yieldedness creates hopelessness. Brokenness can be the effect of a passive reaction to a situation. Yieldedness is an active response where we let go and hand over control to God.

'I am crucified with Christ: nevertheless I live; yet not I but Christ liveth in me: and the life which I now live in the flesh I live by the faith of the Son of God, who loved me, and gave Himself for me.' **Galatians 2:20**

- **Will to be the best**

Right choices are righteous choices and righteous choices are right choices (Matthew 6:33). When you make the right choice there is peace, joy and faith even if it may be a difficult circumstance (Matthew 5:10). Right choices bring right outcomes. Daniel made the right choice, which was a righteous choice when he could have accepted what was on offer (Daniel 1). He was 10 times wiser because he didn't settle for second best. Not all right choices in the world's eyes are righteous choices in God's eyes, e.g. abortion.

- **Discipline decides**

Discipline is a deciding factor between destiny and destination. Disciplined people bring destiny to its destination. A disciplined will is a vital part of godliness. Ants rule the undergrowth by their discipline and order (Proverbs 30:25).

'Brokeness is the product of the realisation that you can't do it yourself and you need God. You can then yield to God. Yieldeness with out brokenness is only psychology and has no power.'

(10 minutes)

1. **What influences the choices you make in life?**
2. **What areas of discipline and time management do you need to improve?**
3. **Do you compromise quality for quantity?**

Personal *Thoughts*

SECTION FOUR - HEALTH OF THE BODY

CHAPTER SIX

FOOD: THE STAFF OF LIFE

A. EAT TO LIVE, DON'T LIVE TO EAT

Food is good, the Bible says (Genesis 1: 12,30,31). Food is as necessary to our bodies as the air we breathe and yet when did you last see an "oxygen addict" or a diet for reducing the air we breathe? Food is a basic necessity – "the staff of life" so bread is called, and yet it evokes so much more of a response in us than air or water. Food has taken on a whole new meaning due to cookery programmes, chef superstars, restaurant culture and the recent global phenomenon of diets such as the Atkins Diet.

1. Food as a relationship

As Eve found out in the Garden of Eden – it isn't just the food and its taste that can be damaging but the role that food plays in our life. Eve found out to her detriment that not all that looks nice is nice!

Obesity is a global epidemic with increasing urbanisation in developing countries. There is a reduction in physical activity as people live in a computer age with long working hours and little exercise and more processed fast foods. We now eat less fat than at the end of the 19th Century but increasing amounts of sugar, salt and simple carbohydrates. This is creating an epidemic of western diseases such as diabetes and heart disease. Even in developing countries where there is urbanisation of the population they are seeing rising incidences of heart disease and diabetes. The western world has 23 per cent of adults being obese and 30-50 per cent being overweight. Tragically, the future looks bleak, as 5-15 per cent of children are now overweight.

When Eve picked the fruit (Genesis 3:6), not only did she die spiritually but she also suffered rejection and fear. She was damaged emotionally and psychologically.

Her body image was distorted as shame took its strangle hold upon her. From being naked and NOT ashamed, she became naked AND ashamed. Separated from God, she was riddled with guilt and condemnation, no longer able to receive love or experience intimacy. Food that was good became a point of contact for the enemy to damage her emotionally and spiritually. It even affected her marriage as intimacy and trust was lost between her and her husband. It wasn't that food was suddenly bad. It was still good, as God had declared. It was her RELATIONSHIP with food and the role it took in her life that became the stumbling block.

1-2 percent of women are now anorexic with a distorted body image to the point of delusion where they can literally starve themselves to death; 5-10 per cent experience bulimia with binge eating followed by self-induced starvation or vomiting.

2. Eating disorders – cause and effect

These are eating disorders with a deeper psychological, emotional and possibly even spiritual root that can be very difficult to treat. Body image has been so grossly distorted that they can no longer accept themselves. Isn't it the same rejection, fear and shame that Eve experienced in the garden? Many eating disorders become evident in teenage years as adolescents struggle for identity and acceptance among peers and friends. They create unrealistic physical expectations for themselves that set a pattern for failure and loss of self-esteem. Food has now taken on a whole new meaning as the child's identity becomes tied to their body image. They love or hate themselves purely on the basis of how they look. As the emotional and hormonal challenges of adolescence develop they can often be compounded by family instabilities, parental divorce and sibling rivalries. Sometimes there can be other very serious compounding factors like sexual abuse and domestic violence that traumatise the child's development.

Eating disorders among men are increasing, as they become victim to the same distortions and challenges of body image that have plagued women for centuries.

Is it possible that the favouritism of Jacob towards Joseph and Benjamin in the book of Genesis led to one of his sons developing an eating disorder? In Genesis 49:20 it tells us that 'Out of Asher his bread shall be fat, and he shall yield royal dainties'. I am sure this could be interpreted in many ways but I wonder if he had a sweet tooth that was taken to extremes. Out of his insecurity there came an iniquity that passed through his generational line of an identity that was tied wrongly to food. Maybe the rejection he felt from his father drove him to comfort eat and find acceptance in food. We may never know for Asher, but I am convinced that rejection is at the root of many emotional problems in men. This could be an increasing contributor to the increase in eating disorders among men.

3. The path to freedom

I am sure Jacob as an imperfect earthly father was not the perfect role model for his sons. I am sure he tried his best and was clearly chosen of God but the consequences of his fallen nature would affect his children. The great truth that we have today is that we don't have to live with the consequences of an imperfect family. God is our Father and through the spirit of adoption the blood of Jesus, claims us as His own and renders the power of the world, the flesh and the devil as nothing. This is the way out for people in these situations. I know from personal experience! I had a distorted relationship with food where it became my relaxation and even my god.

I could easily consume bars of chocolate, a packet of chocolate digestives, all on the back of two to three thick sandwiches and pieces of cake from the West Indian Bakery near my home in north London. I spent many years as a Christian and non-Christian struggling in this area. I could literally not eat for 24 hours and then eat for two hours almost non-stop. Even when I became a "strong" Christian, spirit-filled and winning people to Jesus every week, the problem wouldn't go away. At medical school when I understood the dynamics of food and eating and the psychology around it, it still defeated me.

On one occasion before the Lord, I reflected on how I had overcome all the challenges in my life as a Christian except one, my relationship with food. I couldn't really speak to anyone about it because it seemed so insignificant compared to the weighty matters of heaven and hell!

Food is a safe comfort because it doesn't argue, it doesn't shout back and it is pleasurable. What a friend we seem to have in food. Next to a dog, food is a man's best and worst friend!

Well, instead of God sorting out my food problem He sorted out my 'Liam' problem and laid the axe to the root of the tree. He didn't just prune the fruit, He dealt with the root! My problem wasn't only physical or emotional. It was primarily spiritual. I had all the head knowledge of the unconditional love and acceptance of God as my Father but I had never really experienced it in my heart. My problem wasn't food. My problem was that fundamentally my identity was tied to how well 'I' was doing in my life and as a Christian. If I was full on for God I could overcome my eating problem, but whenever I made a mistake or needed to relax, I would turn to the 'carbs and cakes'. I was living a 'conditional lifestyle'.

The root of 'I', the root of rejection and pride was still resident in me. God brought me to a painful place of complete surrender where the experience of His unconditional love and of the cross became a living reality to me.

Suddenly as I daily yielded my heart to Him, my body no longer ruled my mind. Food was no longer my god and my devil. My will was surrendered and the Holy Spirit became my closest friend. His fruit became my experience - love, joy, peace and self-control. My desires became balanced and nearly 30 years of bondage was broken.

Hallelujah!

> *'My problem wasn't food. My problem was that fundamentally my identity was tied to how well 'I' was doing in my life and as a Christian. I was living a "conditional lifestyle" .'*

Each time I was low or felt the urge to gorge I would pour out my heart to God and yield myself to His control. I found that the strength of the urge would weaken and I would find my fulfilment in receiving His unconditional love for me. It was the genuine article - a deep intimate relationship with God that fulfilled ALL my deepest needs and healed my wounds. My substitute relationship with food became redundant. Over a period of time my lifestyle became spirit, soul and body, in that order, rather than body, soul and spirit in this area.

Many of us live emotions first, or body first and our desires are not under the Lordship of the Holy Spirit. Biblically speaking, we should be spirit first, soul second and body third. If our body is ruled by our senses and our senses by the Spirit then we can experience something of what Adam and Eve experienced before the fall - spiritual, emotional and physical nakedness without shame.

After the Fall, Adam and Eve experienced:

- The spirit - Spiritual death
- The emotions - Dominant negative emotions
- The mind - Lost knowledge of God
- The will - Too many choices
- The body - Physical death

Even if we have experienced much rejection, sexual abuse and shame where our lives are governed by past experiences, I believe there is a place of complete healing and wholeness where we can be naked before God and not ashamed. From this place of strength in God we can have healthy relationships. Isn't that God's promise, 'old things should pass away and ALL things become new' (2 Corinthians 5:17)?

4. The power of food

Henry VIII was known for his voracious appetite; supermodels today for the suppression of it. In an average lifetime a person will eat thirty tons of food! Being such a significant part of our lives, it is no surprise that the enemy would want to do all he can to usurp its influence and make it a stronghold over us. Even the devil's first temptation of Jesus in the wilderness was linked to food (Matthew 4:3). Doesn't this sound familiar to the strategy in the Garden of Eden?

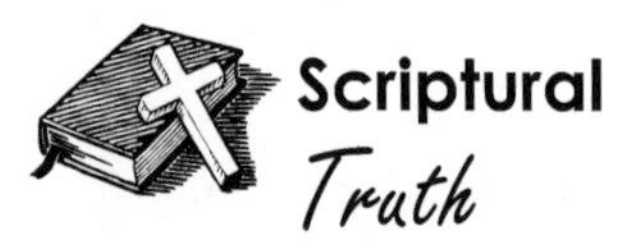

'Now when the tempter came to Him, he said, "If you are the Son of God, command that these stones become bread."' **Matthew 4:3**

The appetite and desire for food is strong and like many things in life, the desire for the wrong kinds of food seems much stronger than the desire for the right kinds.

It requires discipline, wisdom and a life submitted to God to put food in its rightful place. Gluttony and over indulgence is clearly a sin according to scripture and should be dealt with the same seriousness as any other behavioural problem. Jesus used a meal as one the most sacred acts in Christianity. The communion represents the most powerful and holy ceremony we can perform. The very crucifixion of Jesus and all it represents is symbolised in bread and wine. If respect for the cross were the only reason to put food in its rightful place in our lives, it would be reason enough.

B. FOOD AS NUTRIENT

1. Introduction

A healthy attitude and a healthy relationship with food can be both liberating and can be a vital part of walking in divine health. Food provides the bodies building materials for growth and repair and the energy necessary to keep tissues and organs functioning correctly.

Dealing with the emotional and spiritual is important to regulate eating habits. However there are important physical clues to help control and regulate our diets so we can live in divine health. It is not possible for me in the context of this book to do a detailed study of food. My intention is to provide you with some simple principles that you can use to make healthy eating a lifestyle.

2. Food Groups

The basic food groups are protein, fat and carbohydrates. Vitamins and minerals are vital trace elements that are necessary in our diets.

- **Proteins**

Proteins are for muscle building, functioning of enzymes, hormones and other body chemicals.

- **Fats**

Fats are necessary for stored energy, and heat production.

Carbohydrates

Carbohydrates are an important fuel and energy source.

- **Vitamins and minerals**

Vitamins and minerals are important nutrients for the body. They are required for all metabolic processes.

2.1 Proteins

Protein is excellent at stabilising blood sugar to help reduce hunger pains and regulate appetite. People who eat the wrong kind of carbohydrates e.g., cakes, biscuits and foods with a high glycaemia index (see below) in large amounts have unstable sugar levels in their blood stream that can cause cravings, tiredness, fatigue and tend towards binge eating like behavioural patterns. Proteins avoid the insulin surges that create the pattern above.

Increasing lean protein content of a meal (e.g. grilled chicken breast, diced turkey, and fresh fish) is an excellent way of regulating appetite and stabilising blood sugar, thereby helping weight management. It is very hard to eat five steaks but it is quite easy to eat five doughnuts! This is due to the response of the body to the different food groups. Lean protein (avoiding the bone and skin) removes some of the risk associated with some high protein diets, which increase saturated fat content. It is the balance and type of protein, carbohydrates and fats, which are important. 10 - 20 per cent of our diet should come from protein. Preferably fresh fish and lean white meat such as chicken or turkey with limited amounts of red meat.

2.2 Fats

Fat is necessary in our diets. It is the type of fat we eat that matters. Saturated and monounsaturated fats are only used for energy and aren't necessary for life. Polyunsaturated fats or oils are essential. The optimum amount of fat in the diet should be 20 per cent of our total calories. The average in the western world is 40 per cent.

The wrong kind of fats increases our chances of heart disease – the biggest killer of the western world. Polyunsaturated fats include omega 6 and omega 3 fatty acids. There is a lot of publicity about these in the media and they are vital for health.

Omega 6 is linoleic acid, which comes from seeds and their oils e.g., sunflower, hemp, pumpkin, and sesame and Soya bean amongst others. They are also found in evening primrose and borage oil. They are necessary for thinning the blood, immune function, sugar balance and reducing inflammation.

Omega 3 is alpha-linolenic acid (DHA and EPA). These are found in flaxseed (linseed), pumpkin and hemp seed oil. They are also found in oily fish-mackerel, herring, tuna and salmon. They are important for blood thinning, blood fats, immune function, water balance, reducing inflammation and for brain function. The ideal ratio of the above in our diet is 2:1, omega 6:omega 3. In reality most of the western diet is deficient in both so we had better get used to eating oily fish and seeds! It is particularly deficient in omega 3.
WARNING – pregnant women should not eat more than 1 portion of tuna a week due to the possible mercury levels present.

'The olive oil story'

Olive oil is as old as man can remember. Although the amount of omega 3 and 6 is not great, the quality of olive oil is due to its unrefined nature, which makes it a purer source of healthy fats than other, refined vegetable oils like sunflower oil. Extra virgin olive oil is the best. It is mainly a monounsaturated fat. Saturated (hard) fats are mainly the red meat and dairy products. A high intake of these is definitely associated with heart disease.

Margarine is classified as a polyunsaturated fat and therefore apparently healthy. The problem is in its refining and processing. It has been through a process called hydrogenation, which converts it into a trans fat. This process does two things. Firstly, it blocks the body's ability to use other healthy polyunsaturated fats.

Secondly, it releases toxic free radicals that damage body cells and tissues. Frying has the same effect on oils as the above and should be avoided.

To make up the 20 per cent of our diet that should be fat, we should have 5 per cent omega 6 fats (evening primrose oil and seeds), 3 per cent omega 3 (seeds and oily fish), 7 per cent monounsaturated (olive oil) and 5 per cent saturated fat (meat and dairy).

2.3 Carbohydrates

This is a developing science. We are beginning to understand more about carbohydrate metabolism and its relationship to insulin.

The Glycaemic Index (GI) is a simple mechanism to help you eat the right kinds of carbohydrate in your diet. A food with a high GI (>70) will cause a lot of sugar to be released into your blood stream quickly. This gives you an initial energy boost but also causes a large amount of insulin to be released, emptying the blood stream of that sugar. This causes the blood sugar level in the bloodstream to drop and can cause an energy dip amongst other symptoms. You then take more sugar to increase your energy again. This cycle of highly fluctuating levels of sugar can eventually lead to an inability of the insulin to mobilise the blood sugar and can eventually lead to diabetes.

These fluctuations in sugar and insulin levels can lead to cravings and binge eating particularly if food is used for comfort. Insulin regulates fat metabolism and a diet dominated with the wrong kind of carbohydrate can rapidly lead to weight gain even if the quantity of food doesn't seem to be great. This is the frustration of many a dieter. Insulin is also important in fat metabolism by reducing breakdown of fat and storing excess sugar as fat.

Eating the right kind of carbohydrates is very important. Having a diet with predominantly lower GI foods (below 50) will help to regulate blood sugar and breakdown fat when coupled with an active lifestyle. (See below 'Check list of Glycaemic Index rating'). The Glycaemic Load (GL) takes this to another level. It includes the GI but adds in the concentration of a particular carbohydrate in food as well as its sugar release.

An excellent pocket guide to GL is available through a nutritional company called Higher Nature (see Bibliography).

Simple sugars

These need minimal digestion and enter the bloodstream quickly. They include white and brown sugar, glucose (in chocolate bars and Lucozade), honey and syrup. Fruit and milk products are simple sugars but are released slower into the body because they must be converted into glucose.

Complex sugars

These are more slowly digested and include:

- Starches (polysaccharides) – vegetables, lentils, grains beans and potatoes.
- Fibre (indigestible polysaccharides) – the fibre part of starches. The more complex carbohydrates we have the better our blood sugar is regulated. This helps to regulate appetite, bowel function, reduce hunger pains and increase vitamin and mineral content of our food.

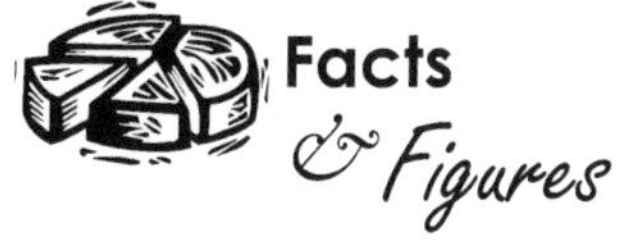

Glycaemic Index:

Item	Value
Glucose	100
Maltose	100
Lucozade	95
Honey	87
Mars Bar	68
Sucrose (house hold sugar)	59
Fructose (fruit sugar)	20

Fruit

Item	Value
Raisins	64
Bananas	62
Orange juice	46
Oranges	40
Apples	39

Grains

Item	Value
Brown bread	72
White bread	69
Granary bread	46
Rye bread	65
White rice	72
Brown rice	66
Basmati rice	58
Rvyita	69
Pastry	59
Digestive biscuits	59
Rich tea biscuits	55
Oatmeal biscuits	54
Sweet corn	59
White spaghetti	50
Wholemeal spaghetti	42
Pasta	40-60

Cereal

Item	Value
Cornflakes	80
Weetabix	75
Shredded wheat	67
Muesli	66
All Bran	52
Porridge oats	49

Pulses

Item	Value
Baked beans (no sugar)	40
Butter beans	36
Chick peas	36
Black eyed peas	33
Haricot beans	31
Kidney beans	29
Soya beans	15
Lentils	29

Diary Products

Item	Value
Ice cream	36
Yoghurt	36
Whole milk	34
Skimmed milk	32

Vegetables

Item	Value
Cooked parsnips	97
Cooked carrots	47
Instant mashed potatoes	80
New potatoes	70
Cooked beetroot	64
Peas	51

40-60 per cent of our diet should consist of carbohydrates. With the major content of our diet being carbohydrate we can see why the right choices here can make a significant difference to our overall health and weight control.

If we build our diet around whole food, raw, fresh and organic carbohydrates we will have a healthy balance of energy, sugar regulation and nutrition to live an optimum lifestyle in divine health. Evidence shows that the Mediterranean diet is the healthiest that has been studied. This protects us against heart disease and is very close to the Biblically- prescribed diet in the Old Testament. It is no surprise that the God who created the world also knows how to live in the world! The Mediterranean diet is high in olive oil, seeds, fruit, vegetables and fish. While we are free to eat all kinds of food other than things strangled, offered to idols and blood (Acts 15: 29),it is also our responsibility to look after our bodies in the best way we can. They are the temples of the Holy Spirit (1 Corinthians 6:19-20).

3. Food and the Bible

The Bible has many references to food and I have tried to summarise some of the key dietary principles below. These are not laws but guidelines as under the new covenant of grace we are free to choose what we eat. However, many of the Old Testament references regarding food and eating came direct from God and it would seem wise to take heed. Many of these guidelines have been scientifically validated and clearly demonstrate God's detailed interest in how we care about ourselves physically as well as spiritually.

- **Avoid saturated fat**

This kind of fat is high in the wrong kind of cholesterol (LDL cholesterol). It lies in the wall of arteries where it forms plaques. This increases the risk of heart disease and strokes.

'It shall be a perpetual statute for your generations throughout all your dwellings, that ye eat neither fat nor blood.' **Leviticus 3:17**

'Speak unto the children of Israel, saying. Ye shall eat no manner of fat, of ox, or of sheep, or of goat.' **Leviticus 7: 23**

- **Eat the right kind of fats**

Olive oil, olives and fats from seeds and nuts.

'houses full of all good things, which you did not fill, hewn-out wells which you did not dig, vineyards and olive trees which you did not plant - when you have eaten and are full.'

Deuteronomy 6:11

- **Eat whole grains**

These help to lower cholesterol, increase fibre content of the diet and have a higher nutrient content.

'And God said, "See, I have given you every herb that yields seed which is on the face of all the earth, and every tree whose fruit yields seed; to you it shall be for food". ' **Genesis 1:29**

'A land of wheat and barley, of vines and fig trees and pomegranates, a land of olive oil and honey.' **Deuteronomy 8:8**

- **Eat plenty of fruit**

Contains fruit sugar, which regulates blood sugar better (e.g. for diabetics) and is high in fibre, which lowers cholesterol and improves bowel function.

'And every tree whose fruit yields seed; to you it shall be for food.'
Genesis 1:29

- **Avoid uncooked meat**

Although this verse refers specifically to kosher food it does raise the issue of blood and the importance of blood borne diseases that can be carried in meat that isn't cooked sufficiently.

'It shall be a perpetual statute for your generations throughout all your dwellings, that ye eat neither fat nor blood.' **Leviticus 3:17**

'That ye abstain from meats offered to idols, and from blood, and from things strangled, and from fornication: from which if ye keep yourselves, ye shall do well.' **Acts 15:29**

- **Eat the right kind of fish**

They are included in Leviticus 11:9 as a part of 'everything in the waters'. The clean ones according to the Bible are those with fins and scales. This avoids the scavenging type of seafood like crustaceans, shellfish etc, which have a higher disease load, unless cooked correctly. Also the scales of fish collect the heavy metals like mercury, which can then be removed easily. Shrimps and shellfish retain heavy metals in their flesh.

- **Eat the right kinds of meat**

The scripture teaches to avoid scavenging birds, reptiles (Leviticus 11:29-30), all insects except grasshoppers (Leviticus 11:21) and only to eat mammals that are ruminants (chew the cud) such as cows that have cloven hooves (Leviticus 11:7). The main one of exclusion is the pig. It is well known that this animal is a scavenger and carries more diseases than many other animals.

It is very important to remember that we are under a covenant of grace and the above are guidelines and not laws. The New Testament clearly teaches that we shouldn't offend our brother and we should walk in love being grateful for any food that is placed before us while avoiding that which is strangled, offered to idols and blood (Acts 15: 29).

'For it seemed good to the Holy Spirit, and to us, to lay upon you no greater burden than these necessary things: That you abstain from things offered to idols, from blood, from things strangled, and from sexual immorality. If you keep yourselves from these, you will do well.' **Acts 15:28-29**

Many of the Old Testament festivals were built around food as a part of the social and spiritual exercise. Jesus' ministry often involved meals. Food is a powerful force for good as it encourages social interaction and service to one another.

4. Food as a diagnosis

The following is a checklist of questions to ask yourself which could reveal an eating or food - related problem:

Carbohydrate problem

- Do you need a cup of tea, coffee or something sweet in the morning to get going?
- Do you often feel drowsy or sleepy during the day or after meals?
- Do you fall asleep in the early evening or need naps during the day?
- Are you rarely awake within twenty minutes of rising?
- Do you avoid exercise because you do not have the energy?
- Do you get dizzy or irritable if you go six hours without food?

- Is your energy level less than it used to be?
- Do you get night sweats or frequent headaches?

If you answer yes to more than four then you probably have problems in regulating your blood sugar level.

Fat problem

- Do you have high blood pressure?
- Do you suffer from premenstrual syndrome, water retention or breast pain?
- Do you suffer from eczema, dry skin or dry eyes?
- Do you have any inflammatory health problems like arthritis?
- Do you drink alcohol every day?
- Do you have difficulty losing weight?
- Do you have a blood sugar problem or diabetes?
- Do you have problems with memory and learning?
- Do you have excessive thirst?

If you answer yes to more than five you may have a deficiency of omega 3 or omega 6 oils.

Eating disorder:

- Are you never happy with the way you look?
- Do you deflect compliments about how you look?
- Do you ever make yourself sick because you feel uncomfortably full?
- Do you ever worry you have lost control over how much you eat?
- Have you ever lost more than 1 stone over a 1-month period?
- Do you believe yourself to be fat when others say you are thin?
- Would you say that food dominates your life?

If you answer yes to three or more of the above you may have an eating disorder.

IT IS VERY IMPORTANT THAT IF YOU FEEL YOU HAVE AN EATING DISORDER THAT YOU SPEAK TO SOMEONE YOU TRUST. DON'T KEEP IT TO YOURSELF. YOU WILL NEED HELP BOTH PERSONALLY AND PROFESSIONALLY. I ADVISE THAT YOU SHOULD DISCUSS THIS WITH YOUR DOCTOR AS SOON AS POSSIBLE.

5. Food in summary

- Eat smaller regular meals, i.e. 3-5 meals a day. Avoid skipping meals, large meals or bingeing and eating too late at night
- Eat 5-7 portions of fresh fruit and vegetables a day
- Have a 3:1 ratio of non-tropical fruit e.g., apples, pears or citrus fruit, to tropical e.g., bananas, pineapples, kiwi
- Have a 3:1 ratio of green leafy vegetables e.g. spinach, broccoli and cabbage, to legumes, lentils and root vegetables such as potatoes, parsnips and carrots
- Eat fresh fish e.g. salmon, mackerel and herring, and lean white meat. Limit red meat to twice a week
- Eat 7-10 fresh nuts a day e.g. almonds, Brazil nuts and walnuts. Use these as alternative snacks or in homemade muesli
- Eat seeds as a snack, on cereals or salad. Flaxseed 1-2 dessert spoonfuls sprinkled on cereals or pumpkin seeds on salad
- Eat low fat dairy products and consider Soya milk instead of cow's milk, particularly if you have a dairy intolerance
- Eat organic foods as much as possible to reduce contamination with hormones, pesticides and antibiotics. Especially for meats, dairy products, potatoes, tomatoes, bananas, sultanas/raisins, apples, lettuce and strawberries
- Try Soya (tofu), beans, lentils and quinoa as a source of vegetable protein to replace animal protein

- Avoid frying; stir fry with olive oil if doing any frying. Steam vegetables as lightly as possible. Microwaving and excessive boiling can reduce the nutrient content significantly
- Eat whole grains. Rye, granary and multigrain breads, oats, wholemeal pasta and brown rice or basmati rice are best. Consider making homemade muesli for breakfast made from raw ingredients
- Have a high fibre diet from whole grains, fruit, vegetables, oat bran, wheat bran, nuts and seeds
- Avoid sugar, refined and white foods. Use fructose (obtained from supermarkets or health food shops) instead of sucrose (household sugar) for sweetener
- Be adventurous. Buy a bread maker and juicer to use the raw ingredients that you know!
- Limit tea and coffee to 2-3 cups a day maximum, as they will affect your blood sugar balance. Replace with herbal or fruit teas
- Remember what you eat on a regular basis
- What is your lifestyle eating habit?

With the above you will feel healthier, have more energy, balance your blood sugar for better weight control - and you can have the occasional treat without feeling guilty! Eating right will reduce your risk of many diseases including diabetes, heart disease, certain cancers and many digestive problems.

Eating the right foods, in the right way, at the right time is a critical part of a healthy relationship with food as it reinforces the right patterns of appetite, self-control, lifestyle habits and nutrient balance that will cause you to be free from and free to - free from the power that food may have over your life, and free to eat as God intended you to - without guilt and without gluttony! This way you will win the battle of the bulge and the battle of the binge.

Eating the right foods, in the right way, at the right time is a critical part of a healthy relationship with food. It re-enforces the right patterns of appetite, self control, lifestyle habits and nutrient balance that will cause you to be free from and free to eat

We are what we eat and we eat what we are. It is true to say that in many ways 'we are what we eat', but it is also true to say that 'we eat what we are'. How we feel, how we see ourselves, how we've been brought up, and how society has portrayed food will all influence how and what we eat. How many times have we sat in a city centre watching people go by. As an overweight child passes by – lo and behold an overweight adult follows, or vice versa. Rationing in the Second World War produced a nutritionally, relatively healthy, non-obese population of those who survived. They were clearly a product of their environment, albeit a very sad one. Microwave meals and convenience foods have revolutionised the way we eat. However, for some people food takes on a whole new meaning - a comfort in depression, a source of happiness when all around us is sad; a pick me up when life becomes stressful, or even an overwhelming preoccupation that dominates our lives like an ever-present nightmare. How do we deal with this? Some of these relationships with food are hormonal, some are a natural part of life; but some a dangerous cancer that eats away at our spiritual, emotional and physiological health.

In these cases it is so important that we 'face the music'. Identify the real root of the problem and if necessary get help. Eating for emotional or spiritual support is often a hidden behaviour but it can be as powerful as any other addiction like gambling, smoking or alcoholism and needs to be treated just as seriously. Recognising that God wants to help you in it is important-God came looking for Eve while she was hiding.

God is longing to restore intimacy, remove guilt and shame and bring wholeness. The beginning of this is to recognise God's unconditional love and acceptance. Your cyclical habit of success and failure in your relationship with food can cloud your vision of His unconditional grace. Grace is reflected in the ability to receive what is not rightfully yours and as you hear the words 'you are my beloved son (or daughter) in whom I am well pleased' you can receive the grace to turn to God and not to food. As this becomes a daily dependence, IN your pain, IN your need, IN your habit then the power of the law of sin and death, the pull of the flesh and the patterns of the old can be broken and a genuine fulfilment of your heart and desire in Him can take place. This will not be immediate. For many an eating pattern has been established for a long time. If at a basic level you can come into an unconditional relationship with food that results from an unconditional relationship with God then you are on the road to recovery and healing. After you invite the Holy Spirit to rule this area of your life, yield to His self-control and guidance, allow His 'yes be yes' and 'no be no' food will be removed from the primary focus of your life. Follow this by eating the right foods in the right way at the right time and you'll be able to say 'my body IS the temple of the Holy Spirit'!

My motto is 'eat when I am hungry, drink when I am dry and if God doesn't take me I'll live till I die!'

'*Therefore, whether you eat or drink, or whatever you do, do all to the glory of God.*' **1 Corinthians 10:31**

'*Be anxious for nothing, but in everything by prayer and supplication, with thanksgiving, let your requests be made known to God. And the peace of God, which surpasses all understanding, will guard your hearts and minds through Christ Jesus.*' **Philippians 4:6-7**

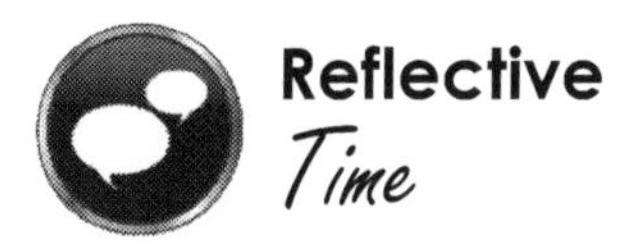

Reflective *Time*

(1 week)

1. **Write down a diary of one week's eating habits and compare it to the above guidelines**
2. **How regularly do you sit down and have a meal with your family?**
3. **What three things could you do to improve your eating habits?**

Personal *Thoughts*

CHAPTER SEVEN

WATER: THE FOUNTAIN OF LIFE

Introduction

'That he might sanctify and cleanse it with the washing of water by the word.'
Ephesians 5:26

There are four very important issues related to water:

1. It is the most important physical substance for life on the planet
2. It can exist in a solid, liquid and gas state depending upon environmental conditions
3. Three quarters of the earth's surface is covered by water
4. More than 70 per cent of our physical make up consists of water

It is no surprise then that water is used in the bible to signify the two most critical elements in the universe - the Spirit (God is a Spirit - John 4:4-14) and the Word of God (Ephesians 5:26).

1. Benefits of Water Intake

- Detoxification - It cleanses and prevents toxic build up
- Hydration (see below)
- Metabolism - water is necessary for the body's metabolic processes
- Dehydration

Five percent of Americans are chronically dehydrated. This can cause fatigue, poor skin condition, dizziness, headaches, reduced concentration and short-term memory. Mild dehydration can reduce metabolism by 3 per cent.

2. Water Excess

There is a definite trend towards water drinking and bottled water is big business. There is a balance as too much water isn't good.
High water intake alters the mineral balance including excess sodium loss. With

excessive intake it can lead to a heart attack particularly if combined with recreational drugs like ecstasy.

3. Types of water

Tap water

- Must pass 57 tests for contaminants
- May have higher European Standards for quality than bottled water
- Some toxic and chemical elements are not removed
- May lack some of the trace mineral content of bottled spring water
- Treated with chlorine to reduce pathogens
- Fluoride added in some areas – controversial. Fluoride is claimed to reduce dental caries. Fluoride as an element is highly toxic

Bottled water

- Must pass 15 tests for contaminants
- Higher mineral content from flowing through natural rocks. The plastic bottles may contain chemicals including xeno-oestrogens which may affect hormone balance

Distilled water

- Water purified and separated by heating and condensing the vapour. Can lose some of the mineral content

Reverse osmosis

- A process of filtration, which is claimed to maintain absolute purity of the water and remove pollutants
- Requires a special filtration system to be added to your domestic water supply. The domestic filters last approximately seven years
- It is used to remove the salt from salt water to produce fresh water
- It is also used in the food industry, power plants and for maple syrup production

It is recommended that anyone considering using a reverse osmosis filter discuss his or her nutritional management with a doctor or nutritionist who specialises in this area. It is cheaper than distilled water to produce.

Ionized water

This is water that has been 'charged' or has maintained its ionic state. It is claimed that this is the nearest to the state of water within the human cell.

It is claimed to have several benefits:

- Oxygenation
- Alkalinasation
- Hydrogen bonding
- Low surface tension
- Electrical conductivities

Consequently it is claimed to lead to:

- Better absorption
- Improved metabolic function
- Reducing free radicals
- Detoxification

Leading to:

- Disease prevention and improvement
- Longevity of life (15 per cent of Japanese drink ionized water from a water container and have 10 years longer life expectancy than in USA. There may be other factors involved in this difference).

4. Water Tips

- Drink 8 - 10 glasses a day for hydration
- Don't omit salt from the diet completely
- Tea/coffee and fruit juices don't classify as water for ideal hydration (pure water is best)
- Urine that is a light straw colour indicate a correct level of water intake

- People with kidney and thyroid disease may benefit from avoiding fluorinated water as much as possible - (check with your local water authority regarding level and safety of fluoride in your water)
- Fruit juice is the best drink with meals to help iron absorption from food. Drink water between the meals and avoid tea/coffee at meal times as this can block Vitamin C absorption
- Increase water intake with exercise. This particularly applies to short bouts of exercise. A prolonged exercise over 2 hours requires specialist advice due to the danger of water overload (metabolic water)

5. Global Considerations

- 15,000 people die each day as a result of unclean water
- Access to clean water is one of the most cost effective ways of saving lives
- People can survive 40 days without food but can only survive 5 days without water
- Drought is a global killer

Water is truly a fountain of life – whether you filter water, buy bottled water, invest in reverse osmosis or ionizers remember that the use of water and energy conservation are important issues to consider in our global responsibilities. Turning the tap off when brushing our teeth or shaving can significantly cut water usage. With the increasing use of metered water you can save financially by reducing wastage of water consumption.

Closing Thought

'But whosoever drinketh of the water that I shall give him shall never thirst; but the water that I shall give him shall be in him a well of water springing up into everlasting life'. **John 4:14**

Water is symbolised as the Holy Spirit and the Word of God in scripture. This symbolism demonstrates the fundamental importance of water to our life and existence. Without water we cannot survive physically. Without the Word and the Holy Spirit we can exist but not live. Water refreshes, purifies, cleans and invigorates. Spiritually the Word and the Spirit do the same thing. Jesus came to give us life in ALL its abundance. We are not born to die but to live. The Word of God has power to change and transform. The Holy Spirit gives power to live and enjoy life to its full. Natural water is critical for life and health. Spiritually water is critical for total life and total health.

'Natural water is critical for life and health; Spiritual water is critical for total life and total health .'

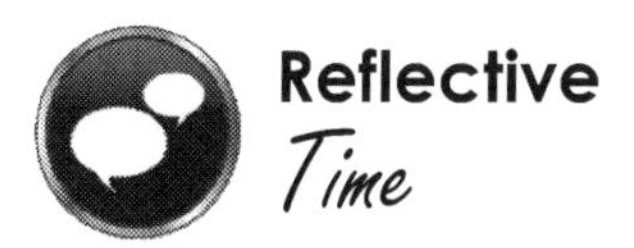

Reflective *Time*

(20 minutes)

1. **How many glasses of water do you drink in an average day?**
2. **How can you conserve water more effectively?**
3. **Have 2 glasses of water between each meal, in the morning upon waking and after each meal. Record how you feel**

Personal *Thoughts*

CHAPTER EIGHT

SLEEP: HELP OR HINDRANCE

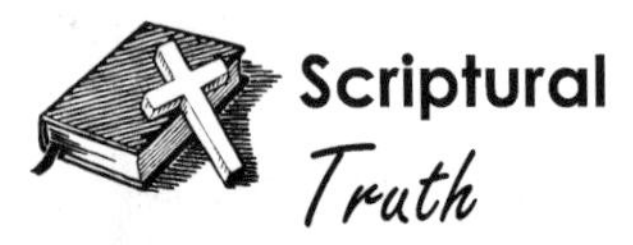

I will both lay me down in peace, and sleep: for Thou, Lord, only makest me dwell in safety.' **Psalm 4:8**

The quality and quantity of our sleep is fundamental to our energy, restoration and function. Recent studies have shown that three half hour naps a week during work hours will lower the risk of heart-related deaths.

There are various reasons why sleep may be important:

1. Reflection – to allow the brain to review and consolidate the streams of information gathered while awake
2. Detoxification – melatonin is the sleep hormone that rises in our body at night and falls when the light shines in the morning. This hormone is one of the most powerful antioxidants (i.e. clears the body of the toxins from normal cell reactions in the body)
3. Refuelling – blood sugar levels drop dramatically after 24 hours of being awake and sugar (glucose) is the brain's fuel
4. Productivity – God put Adam into a deep sleep in order to create Eve and fulfil his need for a helper (Genesis 2:21). Good quality sleep improves our daily productivity
5. Communication – a physical state of rest may be a way in which God chooses to communicate with our spirit through visions and dreams (Acts 10: 9–22)

Sleep is universal among humans and animals. It involves a cycle between two distinct phases: REM (rapid eye movement) and non-REM sleep. It takes 90 minutes to complete a full cycle.

As dawn approaches we spend more time in REM (dreams) sleep. Non-REM sleep has occasional images but REM is where dreams generally occur.
Different frequencies of sleep occur at different times of night and with different ages of a person. This could account for the changes that take place with ageing (tendency to sleep less at night and have a nap in the afternoon).

Sleep deprivation

Sleep is vital to early brain development and function. The average two year old child has spent 18 months of their life asleep.

There is a mindset in certain circles that if you can survive without much sleep you are a role model for all hard workers and achievers. Lack of sleep however doesn't always increase productivity and efficiency. Since 1910 the average duration of sleep has decreased from 9 hours to 7½. Britain was still ruling large parts of the world and truly a global power in 1910 but did so with more sleep per person.

Lack of sleep has been associated with:

- Obesity – due to an appetite-stimulating hormone being increased and appetite suppressants reduced.
- Premature ageing – wrinkling, hair receding, greying.
- Chronic diseases – diabetes, blood pressure, heart attacks.
- Road traffic accidents – up to 30 per cent may be due to driver's sleep fatigue.

Identifying Insomnia and Excessive Daytime Sleepiness

- Insomnia (difficulty falling or remaining asleep) affects up to 25 per cent of the population.
- Narcolepsy (sudden excessive sleepiness) and cataplexy (sudden weakness on emotional arousal).

Epworth Sleepiness Scale

Grade your sleepiness below: -

0 = never doze

1 = slight chance of dozing

2 = moderate chance of dozing

3 = high chance of dozing

Situations

1. sitting and reading
2. watching TV
3. sitting inactive in a public place (e.g. theatre or meeting)
4. as a passenger in a car for 1 hour without a break
5. lying down to rest in the afternoon
6. sitting and talking to someone
7. sitting quietly
8. in a car while stopped in traffic

If your figure is over 11 then there is a high chance of a sleep problem that requires medical attention.

Power napping

This involves short periods of sleep on a regular basis. Some people use this to maintain a round-the-clock lifestyle. Leonardo Da Vinci slept for 15 minutes every 4 hours and survived on 90 minutes sleep a day!

Sleep hygiene

- Sleep long enough to feel refreshed but not more.
- Have regular times of going to bed and waking reinforces the body's natural cyclical sleep-wake rhythm
- Do regular aerobic exercise (not within 2 hours of bedtime)

- Lose weight (obesity can cause Obstructive Sleep Apnoea)
- Avoid temperature extremes in the bedroom
- Alcohol can help people fall asleep but the quality of sleep is reduced causing long-term insomnia
- Resolve issues relationally and mentally. Lack of closure is detrimental to sleep
- Avoid VCRs/TV/Computer 1-2 hours before bedtime
- If you are still awake after 20 minutes get up, leave the room and do a quiet activity before returning
- Hot milky drinks are helpful
- No caffeine (including chocolate/cola/paracetamol) 2 hours before bedtime
- Consult a medical practitioner to resolve any underlying illness such as depression, that can cause early morning waking (EMW) at 3-4am typically

Sleep Remedy

- Resolve underlying issues such as chronic stress anxiety and depression
- Follow the sleep hygiene principles laid out earlier
- Relaxation – finding rest and refreshment for the spirit, the soul and the body is necessary for good quality sleep
- Herbal remedies – can be effective for mild, short-term sleep problems where there is no serious underlying disorder to resolve (e.g. valerian, passion flower). Check with a medical practitioner if you are on medication
- Melatonin – has been used by some people for jetlag, shift work and sleep disturbances. It is an unlicensed medication in the UK. Check with a medical practitioner if you are on medication
- Professional medical help may be required in certain circumstances
- Light boxes – these can be useful in specific medical conditions such as SAD (Seasonal Affecting Disorder) and fibromyalgia

- **Receive His gift of sleeping**

  'For so He gives His beloved sleep.' Psalm 127:2

- **Time management**

  'It is vain for you to rise up early, to sit up late, to eat the bread of sorrows….' Psalm 127:2

- **Cast off burdens**

  'Casting all your cares upon him…' 1 Peter 5:7, Matthew 11:28-30

- **Reflection – biblical meditation**

  'In his law doth he meditate day and night.' Psalm 1:2 Trust God's sovereignty over your life – *'I lay down and slept; I awoke, for the LORD sustained me.'* Psalm 3:5

- **Trust God's sovereignty over your life**

  I lay down and slept; I awoke, for the LORD sustained me.' Psalm 3:5

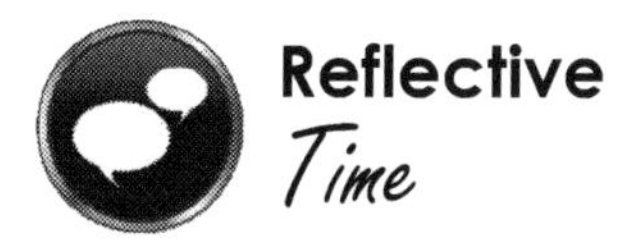

Reflective *Time*

(15 minutes)

1. **Do a sleep diary for 2 weeks including when you went to bed and got up, disturbances in the night, and what you had to eat and drink 3 hours before bedtime**
2. **Do you have excessive daytime sleepiness?**
3. **How do you relax before bedtime?**

Personal *Thoughts*

CHAPTER NINE

LAUGHTER: THE MUSIC OF THE MIND

It is hard to be angry when you are laughing; likewise it is hard to be sad when you are laughing. Laughter is indeed good medicine when it comes from a merry heart (Proverbs 17:22). We need to learn to laugh. Laughter provides a release from everyday responsibilities and challenges. You need to be able to laugh at yourself and with others. We are a peculiar people and human observation can be a humorous pastime. God has created such a diversity of cultures, races and personalities that appreciation of His creation can bring a youthful heart and a lightness of spirit.

Medical effects of laughter are:

- Reduced chronic pain
- Reduced aggression
- Increased mood
- Increased blood flow
- Increased oxygenation of the lungs and removal of waste products
- Boosting the immune system
- Improving relational interaction and bonding

One researcher found that 100 belly laughs a day is an excellent way to get fit.

Society today

People in Great Britain are 'healthier' and richer than at any time in history. Surveys have revealed that even though we have greater prosperity, people are not happier than 50 years ago. From the 'science of human happiness' there are several key factors affecting happiness:

- Quality of your close personal relationships
- Work situation
- Friends
- Community life

Depression and mental illness closely relates to the statistics for relational breakdown in marriages and in the children of broken families. Two other factors are interesting in relation to happiness. Firstly, a moral life is central to it and secondly, the unhappiest societies that have ever been documented were the atheistic communists. Happiness is a temporary phenomenon but can sometimes come from a real sense of joy from a close personal relationship with God through Jesus Christ. This can happen despite circumstances. Laughter is neither a denial nor an underestimation of real life circumstances and eternal realities. It is, however, recognition that God has the final word on every situation and as humans we need to let go of ourselves at times as a safety mechanism for our health.

It also recognises the fact that humour is a part of God's nature and creation and is intended to be enjoyed and experienced. We live in a world of real suffering but this can become our only focus. At times we need a laughter paradigm where we can take opportunities to *carpe diem* (seize the day). Time with our friends, family, conversations with colleagues and mundane tasks can become creative play when we open ourselves to relationships and innovation. Hobbies can be organised happiness times and free space-time can be a time to discover the 'comedian' within us all.

God created laughter; the devil polluted it (mocking). Godly laughter reinforces relationships, builds people and releases emotion. It is not vindictive, it has no hidden agenda and all can enjoy it. It is one of the few universal languages. If you can help liberate people into laughter it can help them to know that whom the Son has set free is free indeed! (John 8:36)

- **You can laugh in your sorrows**
  'Even in laughter the heart may sorrow, and the end of mirth may be grief.' Proverbs 14:13
- **You can laugh with relief and surprise**
  'And Sarah said, "God has made me laugh, and all who hear will laugh with me." Genesis 21:6
- **You can laugh at impossibility**
- *'Then Abraham fell on his face and laughed, and said in his heart, "Shall a child be born to a man who is one hundred years old? And shall Sarah, who is ninety years old, bear a child?" '*Genesis 17:17
- **You can laugh at calamity**
  'You shall laugh at destruction and famine, and you shall not be afraid of the beasts of the earth. Job 5:22
- **You can laugh at your enemies**
  'He who sits in the heavens shall laugh.' Psalm 2:4
- **You have permission to laugh**
  'A time to weep, And a time to laugh; A time to mourn, and a time to dance;' Ecclesiastes 3:4
- **You can laugh because God is on your side**
  'Blessed are you who hunger now, for you shall be filled. Blessed are you who weep now, For you shall laugh.' Luke 6:21
- **You can laugh until you are full**
  'Then our mouth was filled with laughter, and our tongue with singing. Then they said among the nations, "The LORD has done great things for them." ' Psalms 126:2

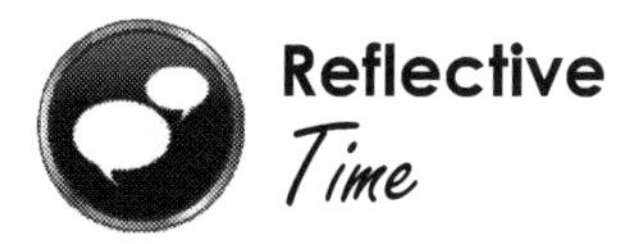

Reflective Time

(15 minutes)

1. **When was the last time you had a good belly laugh?**
2. **What things make you laugh?**
3. **How can you increase laughter in your life?**

Personal Thoughts

CHAPTER TEN

EXERCISE: LOVE OR HATE

'For bodily exercise profits a little, but godliness is profitable for all things, having promise of the life that now is and of that which is to come.'
1 Timothy 4:8

Exercise has temporal value, godliness has an eternal value. Relative to the eternal importance of godliness, exercise is of little importance. However this does not mean that it is of no benefit and indeed exercise is one of the keys to mental, emotional and physical health.

The sedentary lifestyle we now live as a result of computers, cars and a mechanised life is a key factor in the epidemic of obesity we are now experiencing. We have a responsibility to look after our physical body which is the temple of the Holy Spirit (1 Corinthians 6:19). There are many reasons why exercise is important:

1. A Stewardship responsibility before God for the body he has given us
2. Self-respect – if we value what God has given us it will be natural for us to want to look after it
3. Structure – it is the temple of the Holy Spirit and is necessary for God to inhabit our lives on earth
4. Spiritual discipline – physical discipline of our bodies through exercise often reflects a life that is disciplined spiritually. The Methodist Revival of the 18th century emphasised the reflection of spirituality upon our physical discipline and self-control
5. Vitality – exercise improves posture, endurance and mental capacity
6. Physical attraction – Adam was attracted to the physical condition of Eve as well as the spiritual and relational union (i.e. bone of my bones, flesh of my flesh – Genesis 2:23). Physical condition and appearance can enhance relational attraction and intimacy. Exercise helps to maintain those aspects

7. Selflessness – if we love God we will want to look after His temple; if we love our spouses we will want to please them physically. If we love people we will not want to depend on others to be responsible for our health due to our own lack of responsibility and consideration. If we love the community, society and nation in which we live we will not want to waste health resources (e.g. NHS). I am speaking about things we can personally take responsibility for. Obesity could bankrupt the health service if it continues at the present rate due to the chronic illnesses it causes. There is a responsibility we have before God, others and creation as to how we care for our physical world
8. Potential – exercise helps to oxygenate our body systems and can invigorate in terms of energy to fulfil our potential spiritually (if you are energised physically you are less likely to sleep during prayer times) and personally (your capacity for daily things increases and your quality of sleep improves)

Jesus had a physical job (carpentry), walked long distances and was physically fit.

Health Benefits

- Pain relief – due to the release of pain killing chemicals endorphins and encephalins
- Mood boosting – as above
- Strengthens bones
- Regulates blood sugar – lowers the risk of diabetes
- Reduces the risk of breast cancer and colon cancer
- Reduces blood pressure
- Slows down the ageing process
- Improves circulation, muscle and skin tone
- Waste elimination through perspiration (there are 96 million pores in the body)

How?

Be creative and link exercise to things you enjoy (e.g. power walking in the park). Listening to music can be helpful for some people while doing exercise. Doing exercise in groups or in team sports is good for others. Twenty to forty minutes exercise, three to five times a week is what is required. Certain household chores can be included in some of the time periods but specific aerobic exercise like walking or cycling is necessary to improve your heart strength. Remember the heart is a muscle and needs training and strengthening to support its innate rhythm. Resistance exercise such as weights in the gym or weight bearing exercise classes strengthens the bones.

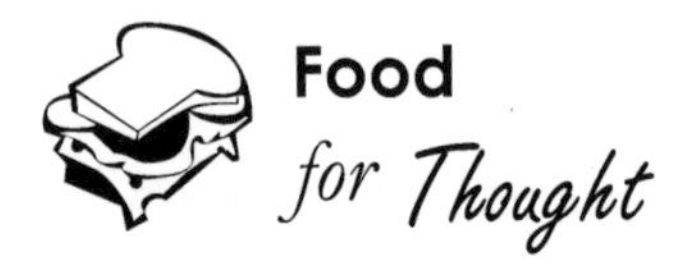

Exercise must be a lifestyle. Summer bursts in the gym will not generate long-term benefits and will be unsustainable. No activity at all is the equivalent of smoking 20 cigarettes a day as far as its health associations are concerned.

Linking exercise to a social focus (e.g. having coffee with an exercise friend afterwards) or family focus (e.g. all going swimming on a Saturday morning) can be helpful. Mobilising a church into exercise can be very productive (e.g. Sunday afternoon football for parents and children can enhance bonding, relationships and evangelistic outreach particularly among men). It is interesting to note that football became a sport of the working classes as a result of the Methodist Reformations. Football was a sport of public schools until the Methodist churches realised that people did nothing after Sunday services as a whole. Because of the Methodist ethos of physical activity encouraging spiritual discipline they mobilised the youth into playing football on Sundays afternoons.

This caught on very rapidly until all over Northern England football became the sport of the masses. That was a vision of biblical social reform directly linked to exercise.

As a rule men overestimate the risk and underestimate what they do. Lack of exercise is a silent killer of the 21st century generation. God gave Adam a garden to enjoy but also to share with his wife. He was commanded by God to dress it and keep it. There was a physical activity, which was pleasant, social, relational and spiritual as God walked with Adam in the garden. After the fall physical activity in the garden became a chore as thorns and thistles began to grow. We cannot stop the thorns and thistles but in redemption we can try and make the garden fun again.

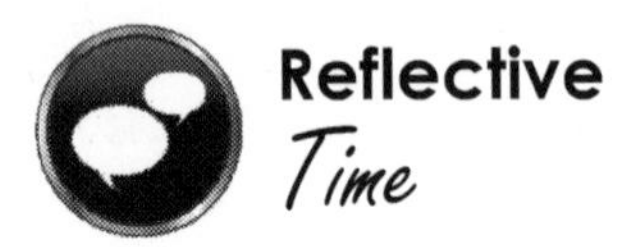

(15 minutes)

1. **How much physical activity do you get in 1 week?**
2. **What is stopping you from doing more exercise?**
3. **How can you increase regular physical activity?**

CHAPTER ELEVEN

FASTING: PLEASURE OR PAIN

'I humbled my soul with fasting'. **Psalm 35:13**

Fasting seems an unusual act of spiritual and physical activity. It is rarely spoken about in conventional medical circles and often neglected in church life. The spiritual reasons and purposes of fasting are many of which this manual has not the scope to deal with in detail. The spiritual and physical acts of fasting reinforce each other. I have highlighted a few below.

Health benefits

It has been suggested that fasting creates the ideal conditions for the body to self regulate, strengthen its immune system, heal itself and channel its biochemical energy used for food and digestion to be used for repair, restoration and disease control.

Benefits include:

- Elimination of toxins
- Slow the ageing process
- Heighten mental alertness
- Clarity of senses and emotions
- Physiological rest of the body for regeneration

Fasting is mentioned 74 times in the Bible and is one of the oldest forms of health therapy. It is not a physical cure within itself, no more than the physical act of fasting can twist God's arm about a specific issue. It may provide the right conditions for the body's own mechanisms of repair, regeneration and revitalisation to take place. Spiritually, it also helps to provide the right environment for focus, relationship and clarity that helps us to keep centred on God.

For health benefits the key to fasting is regularity. In the early stages of fasting (day 1-3) there are often physical symptoms such as headaches from caffeine withdrawal, tiredness from temporary falls in blood sugar, etc. These pass and become easier to deal with when we fast regularly.

- **An act of obedience**
  Then shall they fast...' Luke 5:35
- **An expected spiritual discipline**
  'When you fast...'(not if you fast) Matthew 6:16
- **A focus on God and spiritual issues**
  'I proclaimed a fast there' Ezra 8:21
- **A personal consecration**
  *'I humbled my soul...'*Psalm 35:13
- **A practical purpose**
  *'Is this not the fast that I have chosen?'*Isaiah 58:6-8
- **An act of devotion**
  *'And I set my face unto the Lord God... with fasting'*Daniel 9:3
- **An act of power**
  *'kind goeth not out but by prayer and fasting'*Matthew 17:21

'Fasting may provide the right conditions for the conditions for the body's own mechanisms of repair, regeneration and revitalisation to take place. Spiritually, it helps provide the right environment for focus, relationship and clarity that helps us to keep centred on God .'

There is always a cautionary note in relation to fasting. If a person has a specific medical problem or is pregnant then the person should seek medical advice before embarking upon a fast.

Types of fasting

- Absolute fast – water only
- Total fast – no food or water
- Partial fast – variations of fasting including omission of certain foods, meals and activities. The modern trend of abstaining from certain activities as a form of fasting is a variation on fasting. Strictly speaking the word 'fast' relates to absence of food and/or drink. Stopping certain activities for spiritual purposes is an abstaining or omitting as opposed to fasting. It can still however be a powerful discipline.

Practical guidelines

I prepared a guideline for my previous senior minister who was conducting a 40-day absolute (water fast). On completing the fast I asked him several months later to highlight certain points that were helpful and I thought they were particularly relevant. They were:

- Be sure God is in the fast and not just your own desire
- Fast with medical supervision
- Begin the fast slow – don't cut off all foods at once
- Stop meats and other high protein foods first and a day or so later cut out solids
- Finally eat some fresh soft fruits before the total fast
- Keep fluid intake high throughout the fast – pure water
- Be prepared for days of high toxic breakdown – these leave you lethargic
- Conserve energy throughout the fast – do not exert yourself
- Keep a record of weight loss and know danger signals of muscle and organ wastage

- Watch for the return of hunger pains between 3-6 weeks – it is dangerous to ignore these as starvation can hit people at different times during this period
- Be aware of the downsides of prolonged fasting – physical weakness, fainting and sleeplessness
- Break the fast when danger signs develop
- Break the fast slowly in reverse order of entering fast – i.e. fluids first, solids and proteins (particularly meat) last
- Build up your physical conditions gradually, exercising until muscle wasting is resolved

It is good to keep a diary of your fast from both the spiritual and physical perspective for your own reflection and future reference of what God showed you or how He answered your prayer.

A practical guideline, if medically appropriate, may be a half-day or one-day fast once a week, a three-day partial or absolute fast once a month, a seven-day partial or absolute fast once a year. The Jewish calendar incorporates regular times of fasting (consecration) and feasting (celebration). A healthy balance of these, with a healthy moderate lifestyle between the regular fasting and occasional feasting, reflects a biblical paradigm of discipline and lifestyle. Fasting was part of the process by which Jesus was led, filled, empowered and anointed by the Holy Spirit. If it was good enough for Jesus then it is good enough for us!

Final thought

'And Jesus being full of the Holy Ghost returned from Jordon, and was led by the Spirit into the wilderness, being forty days tested by the devil. And in those days He did eat nothing: and when they were ended, He afterward hungered.' **Luke 4:1-2**

'And Jesus returned in the power of the Spirit into Galilee, and there went out a fame of Him through all the region about.' **Luke 4:14**

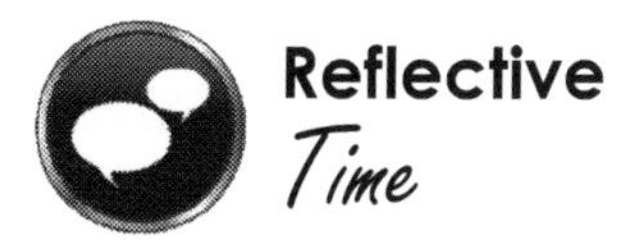

Reflective Time

(15 minutes)

1. **When was the last time you fasted and why?**
2. **How can you incorporate regular fasting into your life?**
3. **Keep a fasting diary of highs and lows and a daily account of response and progress during a fast**

Personal Thoughts

CHAPTER TWELVE

NUTRITION: FACT OR FAD

The modern nutritional state is reflected in a 21st century phrase 'the Affluence Syndrome' which includes the following four aspects:

- Being overfed
- Being undernourished
- A sedentary lifestyle — lack of activity (exercise)
- Chronic stress

This is defined in a specific medical condition that is sweeping the developed world referred to as *Metabolic syndrome* — this is directly correlated to a westernised lifestyle. Its sequelae are as follows:

- Central obesity (being shaped like an apple!)
- High blood pressure
- Insulin resistance (pre-diabetes)
- Inflammation (a marker for heart disease, inflammatory conditions and some autoimmune diseases of ageing)
- High cholesterol

The associations and results of the above are:

- Heart disease and strokes
- High blood pressure
- Obesity
- Diabetes
- Colon cancer
- Alzheimer's disease
- Premature ageing
- Sleep Apnoea

If we do nothing about this we are likely to end up as one of the statistics and possibly die of one of the associations. Drug and medical science can help alleviate some of the issues but will not prevent the syndrome.

Things you can do to stop this:

- Don't smoke and avoid passive smoking
- Regular exercise
- Low GI/ GL diet (see Chapter 6 – Food)
- Low saturated fat diet
- Correct nutrition (see below)
- Address stress

The Metabolic Syndrome is marked by three distinct characteristics of Affluence Syndrome – overfed, under-exercised and chronically stressed. There is an element of under nourishment added to this which affects our immune system.

Functional medicine and nutritional support

1. Why is targeted nutrition important?
2. Is there a place for nutritional supplementation?
3. What is optimum nutrition?

1. Targeted nutrition

This is a huge subject and I can only warrant certain examples below:

Homocysteine levels can be a marker for strokes (amongst other conditions). Homocysteine levels are affected by level of vitamins, folic acid and TMG (Trimethyl glycine). Omega 3 fatty acids in oily fish and certain vegetable oils have been shown to reduce triglyceride in the blood and the clotting of blood. Probiotics (e.g. lactobacillus, acidophilus, bifidobacterium) reduce diarrhoea associated with antibiotics.

Targeted nutrition involves a nutritional treatment being given as a specific therapy. The examples above reflect that.

2. Is there a place for nutritional supplementation?

There is a real and growing controversy over the need for supplementation of our diet. Many foods are picked un-ripened and then transported half way around the world so they can appear a perfect colour and shape on our supermarket shelves. Much of the nutrient concentration in a plant occurs during the ripening stage and is lost when picked too early. We don't yet know the effect of Genetically Modified Food upon nutrition. Soil is intensively farmed with little or no crop rotation and leaving of fallow ground. Fertilisers replenish some of the nutrition but in nature it isn't just the presence of nutrients but how they are combined that is important.

There are several reasons in summary why supplementation may be important:

- Most people do not achieve the necessary dietary guidelines in practice (e.g. 5 portions of fruit and vegetables a day, oily fish once or twice a week and preferably organic and unprocessed food etc)
- Trace element depletion in soils through intensive farming
- Loss of fungi necessary for the plants to absorb trace elements from the soil. Pesticides kill these fungi
- Eating of processed foods. The refining and bleaching process removes much of the nutritional content
- Environmental toxin exposure. Toxins often require vitamins and minerals for excretion from our body. The greater the toxic load the greater the drain on our nutrient status

3. What is Optimum Nutrition?

Deficiency is when the lack of a vitamin or mineral causes symptoms of a disease. It occurs for one of four reasons:

1. Reduced intake (e.g. oily fish is one of the few dietary sources of Vitamin D)
2. Reduced absorption in the gut (e.g. Coeliac Disease affects 1 in 200 of the population. People with this condition are unable to tolerate a certain component of grains)

3. Increased requirements (e.g. exercise, illness)
4. Increased loss (e.g. diarrhoeal illness)

Recommended Daily Allowance of vitamins and minerals is the amount required to prevent disease associated with a deficiency state. The limiting factors in using RDA's as the sole marker for nutritional levels are:

- They do not take into account individual need or variation
- They may not be adequate for optimum health
- They define disease prevention and not health promotion

One person defined the RDA as the 'nutritional equivalent of the minimum wage'.

Optimum nutrition – this is the level of nutrients in the body required to cause organs and systems to work to their maximum potential. To a large degree the optimum nutritional level for an individual will vary and hence we do not have definitive levels for the population. *It is suggested that healing through nutritional therapy can restore the body to a deficiency free state and that health through nutritional therapy restores the body to an optimum state.*

Optimum nutrition is simply giving your body the best nutrients to be as healthy as possible. The individual variation can be based upon genetic strengths and weaknesses, activity, lifestyle, diet and other environmental factors. It is a level of nutrition that promotes optimal mental, emotional, physical and spiritual performance. It is associated with the lowest incidence of ill health and with the longest healthy lifespan.

There are 50 compounds, which have been so far identified as healthy for life. These include fats, proteins (amino acids), minerals, vitamins, carbohydrates (sugars), fibre, light, water and oxygen.

Describing in detail the specifics of an optimum nutritional programme is outside the scope of this book. It is evident however that nutritional support and therapy plays a major role in health in the 21st century.

Recommended Daily Intake of vitamins and minerals:

Nutrient/Vitamin	**RDA**
Thiamin (mg)	1.4
Riboflavin (mg)	1.6
Niacin (mg)	18
Vitamin B6 (mg)	2
Vitamin B12 (mcg)	1
Folate (mcg)	200
Vitamin C (mg)	60
Vitamin A (mcg)	800
Calcium (mg)	800
Phosphorus (mg)	800
Magnesium (mg)	300
Iron (mg)	14
Zinc (mg)	15
Iodine (mcg)	150
Vitamin E (mcg)	10
Selenium (mcg)	No value
Vitamin D (mcg)	5
Sodium (mg)	No value
Potassium (mcg)	No value
Chloride (mg)	No value
Copper (mg)	No value

Nutrients - Benefits & Sources

In the following two pages I have listed the top six foods that contain a particular nutrient and the common sources of these particular sources. Please note that this is not a list of all foods containing that nutrient. The column titled 'benefit' represents the main function of the nutrient.

Nutrient	Benefit	Top six sources	Common sources
Vitamin A	Skin/sight	Liver, carrots, watercress, cabbage, butternut squash, sweet potato	Dairy products, liver, fish, carrot, mango, sweet potato, spinach, broccoli
Vitamin B1	Energy	Watercress, butternut squash, courgette, lamb, asparagus, mushroom	Brown rice, egg yolks, fish, lean pork, milk, whole grains, broccoli, raisins
Vitamin B2	Energy	Mushrooms, watercress, cabbage, asparagus, broccoli, pumpkin	Organic meats, cheese, egg yolks, yoghurt, milk, poultry, green leafy vegetables
Vitamin B3	Energy/blood sugar and cholesterol	Mushrooms, tuna, chicken, salmon, asparagus, cabbage	Organic meats, poultry, whole grains (except corn), nuts, fish, milk
Vitamin B5	Energy/stress hormones	Mushrooms, watercress, broccoli, peas, lentils, tomatoes	Organic meats (liver, kidney), carrots, fish, poultry, milk, nuts, brown rice, beans, bananas
Vitamin B6	Hormones	Watercress, cauliflower, cabbage, peppers, bananas, squash	Cereals, beans, meat, poultry, fish, fruits (bananas), vegetables (potatoes)

Nutrient	Benefit	Top Six Sources	Common sources
Vitamin B12	DNA	Oysters, sardines, tuna, lamb, eggs, shrimp	Milk products, eggs, meat, poultry
Folic Acid	Brain	Wheat germ, spinach, peanuts, sprouts, asparagus, sesame seeds	Leafy green vegetables (spinach, dried beans, peas), cereals, grain products, fruit & vegetables
Biotin	Skin/nerves	Cauliflower, lettuce, peas, tomatoes, oysters, grape fruit	Cheese, organic meats, soy products, eggs, nuts, broccoli, sweet potatoes, oatmeal
Vitamin C	Immune system/ antioxidant	Peppers, watercress, cabbage, broccoli, cauliflower, strawberries	Citrus fruits, berries, vegetables
Vitamin D	Bones-sunlight	Herring, mackerel, salmon, oysters, cottage cheese, eggs	Fatty fish, fish oils
Vitamin E	Antioxidant	Unrefined corn oils, sunflower seeds, peanuts, sesame seeds, beans and peas, wheat germ	Vegetable oils, nuts, green leafy vegetables
Vitamin K	Blood clotting	Cauliflower, brussel sprouts, lettuce, cabbage, beans, broccoli	Dark green leafy vegetables, tea, cheese
Calcium	Bones/muscles	Cheese, almonds, brewer's yeast, parsley, prunes	Dairy products, tofu, dark green leafy vegetables, sardines, salmon, almonds
Potassium	Fluid balance	Watercress, cabbage, celery, parsley, courgettes, radishes	Dried fruit, vegetables, nuts

Nutrient	Benefit	Top Six Sources	Common Sources
Sodium	Fluid balance	Sauerkraut, olives, shrimps, miso, beetroot, ham	Cheeses, canned food
Chromium	Sugar balance/ heart	Brewer's yeast, wholemeal bread, rye bread, oysters, potatoes, wheat germ	Wholegrain products, bran cereals, green beans, broccoli, spices
Manganese	Antioxidant	Watercress, pineapple, okra, raspberries, blackberries, lettuce,	Wholegrains, nuts, leafy vegetables, tea
Magnesium	Energy/muscles	Wheat germ, almonds, cashew nuts, brewer's yeast, Brazil and pecan nuts	Green vegetables, nuts, seeds, fruits, granary bread
Iron	Oxygenation	Pumpkin seeds, parsley, almonds, prunes, cashew nuts,	Meat, fish, poultry, lentils, beans, iron-enriched flours, cereals, grain products
Selenium	Antioxidant	Tuna, oyster, molasses, mushrooms, herring, cottage cheese	Plant foods, some meats, seafood, meats and bread (USA), Brazil nuts, walnuts
Zinc	Immune system/DNA	Oysters, ginger root, lamb, pecan nuts, haddock, green peas	Oysters, red meat, poultry, beans, nuts, dairy products
Bioflavanoids	Antioxidant/ healing	Berries, cherries, citrus fruit	Peppers, buckwheat, grapes, citrus fruit
Choline	Fat metabolism	Lecithin, eggs, fish, liver, soya beans, peanuts	Liver, soya beans, egg yolks, peanuts, cabbage, cauliflower
Coenzyme Q10	Energy/ antioxidant	Sardines, mackerel, pork, spinach, soya oil, peanuts	Sardines, mackerel, pork, spinach, soya oil, peanuts, walnuts
Inositol	Growth	Lecithin, pulses, soya flour, eggs, liver, fish	Cantaloupe, nuts, seeds, rice, beans

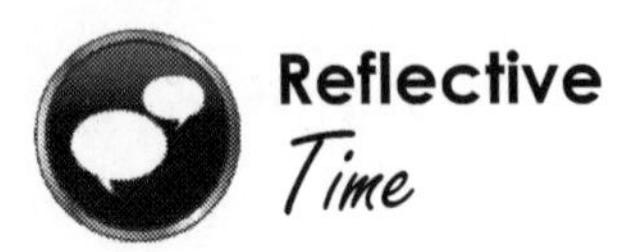

(15 minutes)

1. **How many of the characteristics of Metabolic Syndrome do you have?**
2. **Do you take nutritional supplements and why?**
3. **How can you improve your optimum nutrition?**

Personal *Thoughts*

CHAPTER THIRTEEN

REST: NECESSARY OR NEEDFUL

'Come to me, all you who labour and are heavy laden and I will give you rest.'
Matthew 11:28

Adequate rest is fundamental to productivity and effectiveness. It is estimated that $150 billion is lost to businesses yearly due to fatigue.

Biblical rest encompasses:

- **Silence** - *'Rest in the Lord.'* Psalm 37:7
- **Internal location** – *'Return unto thy rest, O my soul.'* Psalm 116:7
- **Settling** – *'In returning and rest shall you be saved.'* Isaiah 30:15
- **Remaining** - *'There remains therefore a rest for the people of God.'* Hebrews 4:9
- **Ceasing** – *'Sabbath of rest to the Lord'.'* Exodus 35:2
- **Completeness/peace** – *'Neither is there rest in my bones.'* Psalm 38:3
- **Stillness** – *'Rest in the Lord and wait patiently for Him.'* Psalm 37:7
- **Internal state** (to be at rest) – *'Wisdom rests in the heart ...'* Proverbs 14:33
- **Relying upon** – *'Help us O Lord our God, for we rest on You.'* 2 Chronicles 14:11
- **Spiritual place** – *'Clouds rested in the wilderness.'* Numbers 10:12
- **Letting go/releasing** – *'But the seventh year you shall let it rest.'* Exodus 23:11
- **Sleeping** – *'Taking rest in sleep.'* John 11:13
- **Quietness** – *'Rested the Sabbath day...'* Luke 23:56
- **External location** – *'To search out a resting place for them.'* Numbers 10:33

Top tips:

- Let God be God – know your boundaries
- Learn to say no
- Don't feel guilty unless you have reason to be
- Set daily time for reflection and biblical meditation
- Be creative
- Keep a Sabbath for you and your family
- Set time for things that restore you
- Limit access (e.g. telephone, meetings)
- Don't forget fun, friends and hobbies
- Regular exercise, adequate water intake and healthy diet facilitate quality rest
- Find a place to rest. Jesus would go into the wilderness to withdraw and spend time with His Father

'Rest is a good filter to allow your impurities to come to the surface so that you can see things clearly. It opens up free space for creativity, innovation and inspiration.'

These expressions of rest include aspects of willingness, trust, letting go, external place and an internal state. Biblical rest can be very active and powerful as it can involve a place of faith and belief. At other times it is a physical state of inactivity. Rest is necessary for restoration, reflection and renewal. Someone once said that there is more to life than measuring its speed. God can often accomplish more in our rest in Him than in our activity for Him. A survey once asked elderly men what they would change if they could have their life over again. Their response was interesting. They said they would rest more, reflect more and risk more.

Rest is a good filter to allow your impurities to come to the surface so that you can see things clearly. It helps you appreciate life, family and creation. It opens up free space for creativity, innovation and inspiration. Mistakes can often be avoided and true heart feelings identified when we learn how to rest. Life has a certain rhythm and God's creative order has a clock. Early morning is often the time of greatest mental productivity and clarity. It is said that there is a period of stillness within nature between 3am – 5am. Morning devotionals are helpful in setting a 'God' agenda for the day — 'Early will I seek Thee' (Psalm 63:1).

There is a promise of God to respond to those who seek Him early — 'Those who seek Me early shall find Me.' (Proverbs 8:17).

Coinciding with God's creative order, where nature has a high level of activity in the early morning, steady levels during the day and reduced levels in the evening and night (excluding nocturnal creatures!) sometimes helps us dictate our day rather than respond and react to our day. For some there can be a special place that helps facilitate our rest (e.g. sat by a stream, up a mountain or a hill, sat quietly in a rocking chair). Sabbath was made for man and not man for the Sabbath. Rest is required in adequate quantity and quality to live a full and fruitful life.

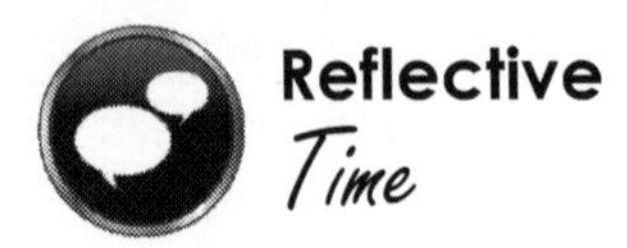

(20 minutes)

1. **How much rest do you have?**
    - **Daily**
    - **Weekly**
    - **Monthly**
    - **Yearly**
2. **What makes you feel rested?**
3. **Diarise and prioritise rest in your life over the next year - *map the gap in your life***

Personal Thoughts

CHAPTER FOURTEEN

STRESS: INEVITABLE OR AVOIDABLE

'Be anxious for nothing, but in everything, by prayer and supplication with thanksgiving, let your requests be made known to God. And the peace of God, which surpasses all understanding, will guard your hearts and minds through Christ Jesus.' **Philippians 4:6-7**

Introduction

What springs to mind when you think of stress? A Type A personality, adrenaline junky, a workaholic person living off caffeine and suffering a heart attack at 45 years of age? Some people say a little bit of stress is good for you. Some can't tolerate even that and avoid any form of stressful situation. Some see stress as a drug that they must have to function. They need a good argument for adrenaline and strong coffee for caffeine first thing in the morning. God is not a masochist. That kind of lifestyle might peak early but die early. I think it is better to peak later and die later. After all Moses peaked at 80 years old and Abraham at 99 years! Jesus is still peaking 2000 years later!

What is stress?

A hundred years ago there was no such word in the English language used in the context of the human condition as understood today. The Compact Oxford English Dictionary defines stress as a *state of mental or emotional strain.*

1. Physical aspects of stress

Physically the body has two main stress hormones. Adrenaline deals with acute sudden stress and cortisol deals with longer-term chronic stress although it can be activated quickly in stressful situations. A small gland behind each kidney called the adrenal gland produces both of these. A third hormone called DHEA, the so-called anti ageing hormone because of many of its actions, is important for protein production. Its level falls with ageing and prolonged stress.

In a shock reaction the body responds by activating these hormones. The body then instigates a counter shock response to balance things again and finally there is an adaptation to the stress. This allows many people to cope with stress for many years. The body is not meant to be under constant stress and hence after a period of time it will begin to show signs of fatigue. The adrenal glands are influenced by wake-sleep patterns, time of day (diurnal rhythm meaning the cortisol and DHEA levels are highest in the morning and lowest at midnight), stimulants such as caffeine and nicotine, and diet such as sugar intake and nutrition.

It is very much a 'lifestyle' organ and responds negatively or positively with time depending upon how we live over many years. I often say that the lifestyle patterns you lay down in your 20's and 30's will determine your health in your 40's and 50's and the lifestyle patterns you lay down in your 40's and 50's will determine your health in your 60's and 70's. This is why so often chronic diseases begin to show themselves in our 60' and 70's such as arthritis, mental illness, heart disease and strokes. The preceding decades of 40' and 50's are often when the signs begin to appear with fatigue, tiredness, obesity, high blood pressure, 'burn-out', depression, mid-life crisis and relationship breakdowns etc. Our body, soul and spirit lifestyle will eventually catch up with us in some way. We are not immune to life and as we will see below I believe that we cannot live stress-free as that is unrealistic but we can seek to live free of the effect of negative stress as that is our goal.

Because we are surrounded by stress doesn't mean we have to be dominated by stress. Some things are genetic and other influences are out of our control. Not every person with the illnesses mentioned above have lived a 'bad' lifestyle. However, there is much we can do to limit the effects of stress on our lives. After all, we were destined to be the 'head and not the tail', 'above and not beneath' as stated in Deuteronomy 28:13. It is interesting that the blessings mentioned in this chapter relate to all areas of our lives, spiritually, occupationally, relationally, nutritionally, parentally, financially, nationally, personally and ministerially. There is a phenomenal blessing of wisdom and wholeness that comes from obedience and intimacy with God.

2. Contributing factors to stress

Our world is always wired, always on-call leaving little room to 'switch off'.

Stress Factors

- Blurring of the lines between work and leisure
- High workloads, lack of control
- Conflict of values between employer and employee
- Relationship and family breakdown
- Lack of spiritual fulfilment
- Stimulant lifestyle – caffeine, nicotine, illicit drugs
- Diet – high processed and sugar loaded foods
- Sedentary lifestyle – lack of exercise
- Low self-esteem – lowers stress resistance
- Hopelessness
- Unrealistic and false expectations

3. Identifying stress

Pressure can be positive and stimulating, i.e. reaching a goal or target. When the pressure exceeds an individual's ability to cope then they are 'under' stress.

- Behavioural changes – losing sense of humour, difficulty making decisions, irritable, poor concentration etc.
- Physical manifestations – diarrhoea, upset tummy, difficulty sleeping, excessive drinking of alcohol.
- Ill health – recurrent infections, chronic tiredness and fatigue, relationship problem, heart disease etc.

4. Stress Checklist

Consider asking your boss to check this list!

- Hard to get up in the morning
- Disturbed sleep patterns
- Tired all the time
- Energy slump in the day
- Feeling weak, muscle and joint aches
- Fatigue
- Faintness
- Craving certain foods
- Obesity around the waist (apple shaped)
- Hungry all the time
- Bloated
- Recurrent infections particularly sore throats
- Poor healing
- Skin spots
- Depression
- Mood swings
- Angry, irritable, aggressive
- Restlessness
- PMT
- Poor memory and concentration
- Difficult to make decisions
- Headache
- Water retention
- Rapid heart beat
- Feeling cold

Many of the above symptoms can indicate other medical conditions and require a consultation with a medical doctor.
Three to five or more of the above may indicate an adrenal hormone imbalance and requires further assessment by a medical doctor.

5. Work Life Balance

Stress costs the economy in the workplace an estimated 5-10 per cent of the gross national product (approx. £3.7 billion a year) and accounts for the largest amount of long-term sickness absence. It is estimated that a ratio of 1:3 workers are so wound up by their job that they can't sleep properly and use alcohol to help relieve stress. Those aged 35-44 were most likely to suffer. Since the Industrial Revolution there have been defining periods with specific characteristics. Innovation and challenging established norms of society epitomised the 1960's. Industrial strife and conflict between employer and employee marked the 1970's. Enterprise associated with alliances-privatisations were typical of the 1980's. The 1990's saw short-term contracts with outsourcing, downsizing and long working hours. Some of these changes led to increased job insecurity, lowered morale and erosion of motivation and loyalty.

A survey of 5,000 British managers on quality of working life found that 81 percent of executives worked longer than 40 hours a week, 32 per cent more than 50 hours and 10 per cent more than 60 hours with some working at weekends.

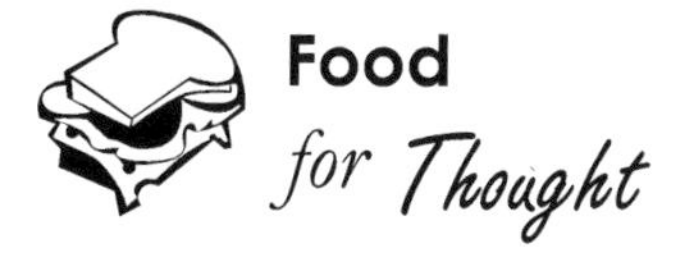

Personal quality of life and economic prosperity are not necessarily the same thing.

A more recent survey over the past five years covering 10,000 managers showed a sustained deterioration in well-being, despite economic growth. Even more worrying was the effect of long working hours on families and health. 56 per cent said it was damaging their health. 54 per cent said it was adversely affecting their relationship with their children and 59 per cent with their partner; 46 percent stated it reduced productivity and 64 per cent claimed that it ruined their social life.

What is clear from this is that the material benefits of modern life and working patterns were having a detrimental effect on the wider scope of a person's life. The purpose of work is not just for financial gain. Some sense of worth and purpose should be a part of the process and integrated into the whole sphere of a person's life. It is better to 'work to live', than to 'live to work'.

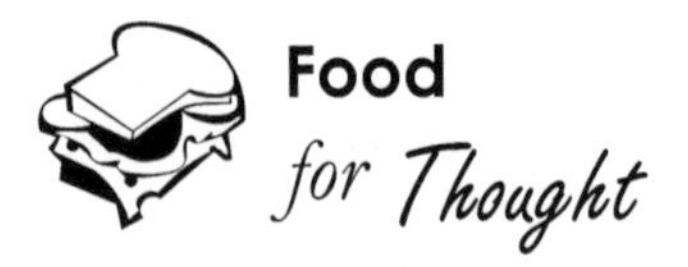

One social anthropologist called Studs Terkel said 'Work is about a search for daily meaning as well as daily bread, for recognition as well as cash, for astonishment rather than torpor, in short, for a sort of life rather than a Monday through Friday sort of dying'

I think there is a lot of truth in that, whether it relates to work, career, ministry or mission. These things are not the ultimate purpose or the end in themselves. They are not worth the sacrifice of our families and futures.

God created the garden for Adam and Eve to dress and to keep. They had a role and work to do but they still heard the voice of the Lord God walking in the garden in the cool of the day (Genesis 3:8). God wanted to meet with them in their daily lives. They were created for God's pleasure and for relationship with Him. If in the process of pleasing and worshipping Him we lose some things of this world then let it be for His glory. Most premature deaths, divorces, diseases and distresses that come from stress and an 'all work and no play' attitude are misplaced loyalties. People are sincere, but sincerely mistaken. Many have missed the fullness of life in experiencing the joys of children, the love of a marriage, the beauty of nature, the simplicity of friendship, the peace of God, the wonder of witness and the rest at work for the sake of an extra pound or a higher role. Promotion is from God, excellence is to be aimed for and hard work is honourable but we mustn't forget that in

Christ all our 'doing' must come from a place of 'being' otherwise we will be at risk of doing it in our own strength.

6. Minimising stress

Primary prevention – Stress avoidance

- Worship, walk and work - in that order
- Live from devotion and not duty first
- Avoid stressful situations – conflict, competition and power struggles
- Plan your thoughts and the day to pre-empt possible pitfalls
- Build teams – some things others can do and others can do better
- Delegate – know your limitations and boundaries
- Don't start what you can't finish. It undermines integrity, generates frustration and de-motivates vision
- Realistic expectations – don't put on you what God hasn't put on you
- Lifestyle is for life. Begin early and follow through to prevent 'burn-out' Don't run too fast too quickly and avoid 'burn-out'. Prevention is definitely better than cure where stress is concerned
- Sleep well, eat right, stay in tune with God's rhythm for your body and avoid stimulants
- Deal with cause not consequence. Internal stress is from you, external from others. Internal rest brings external order
- Don't take yourself too seriously
- Don't take things on board too much – 'burden bearing'

Secondary prevention – Stress management

- What you can't conquer – contain. Some things are for others to deal with but you can avoid the influence
- Maintain what you started under primary prevention
- Balance quantity with quality of life
- Compartmentalise tasks. Deal with things systematically

- Diarise regular breaks before there are no breaks in your diary
- Fix necessities, fulfil needs and enjoy wants
- Know your stress threshold and deal with signs of strain quickly
- God is never overwhelmed – offload often
- Learn to laugh
- Don't change what's not broken. Maximise time management by minimising unnecessary change
- Be content
- Exercise regularly

Tertiary prevention – Stress reduction

- Write down the issues that cause you stress
- Identify the stress factors in your life
- Develop an action plan to change those factors and if they are unchangeable then identify someone who can help you have a different perspective upon them
- Recover what's lost
- If you've broken down, repair. It's never too late to do something. Acknowledge your need
- External help for an internal problem. Don't isolate. Get help
- Communicate clearly
- Relate often. Problem sharing can help problem solving
- God breaks through and not breaks down

7. Health aids for stress

One survey showed that 84 percent of people said that being in contact with nature made them feel more relaxed (any surprise that God put Adam in a garden!).

- Reflection – biblical meditation on God, prayer and faith help to relieve and cope with stress

- Rest – See chapter 13
- Diet – avoid sugar stimulants, excess caffeine, chocolate and alcohol; avoid nicotine and illicit drugs, eat lots of organic fruit and vegetables which counteract some of the inflammatory processes of stress
- Sleep hygiene – see chapter 8
- Exercise regularly – see chapter 10
- Breathing – slower breathing slows down the heart rate and blood pressure
- Nutrition – for the production of stress hormones – adrenalin requires Vitamin B3/B12/C, cortisol requires B5
- Mental well being – glutamine is an amino acid (protein) which is converted to other protein molecules such as GABA which helps 'calm' the nervous system down by regulating other 'feel good' nerve chemicals like noradrenalin, dopamine and serotonin. Glutamine is naturally found in meat, fish, beans and dairy foods. Taurine is another amino acid, which is believed to block the release of adrenalin and 'calm' the system down. It is found in eggs, fish, meat and dairy foods (animal-based)
- Hobbies and holidays – two weeks vacation with no emails can speed reaction time by 82 per cent
- Home life – avoid social isolation. This increases the physiological damage caused by stress
- Have a mission – it helps you to cope with setbacks and disappointments
- Trust God – this helps you find peace, know rest and have hope

Summary

Stress is here to stay. It is a part of 21st century life and living. It doesn't mean, however, that we should resign ourselves to an early grave. Its effect can certainly be lethal and at the very least, prolonged elevated levels of stress can prematurely age us and impair our immune system.

As well as the previously mentioned aids and guides to dealing with this goliath of modern life, Jesus has given us a precious promise of His sustaining presence and victory in this world in which we all live.

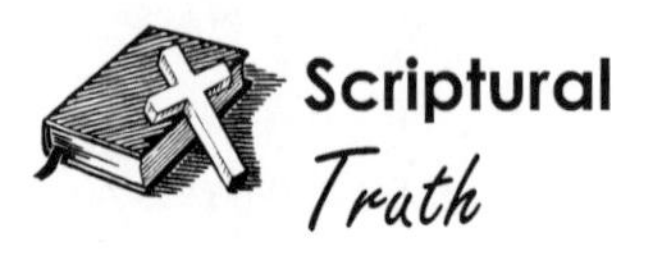

'These things I have spoken to you, that in Me you may have peace. In the world you will have tribulation: but be of good cheer; I have overcome the world.' **John 16:33**

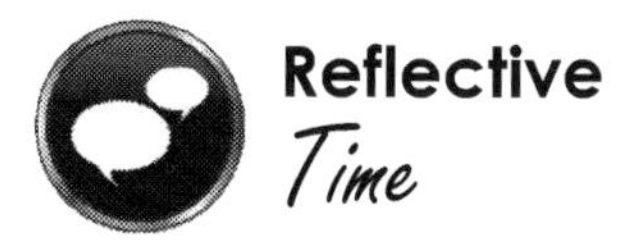

Reflective *Time*

(20 minutes)

1. **How many signs of stress do you have?**
2. **What are the root causes of your stress?**
3. **Where do you want to be in six months in relation to stress management?**

Personal *Thoughts*

SECTION FOUR - HEALTH OF THE BODY

CHAPTER FIFTEEN

MEN'S HEALTH

Introduction

'And God said, Let us make man in our image, after our likeness;...'
Genesis 1:26

What makes a young boy instinctively like trains, trucks and cars? I don't know, other than he is of the male gender. Manhood, maleness and brotherhood are difficult to define but they are a part of a boy's make-up. Not all boys fit the stereotype but there are certain characteristics that make a boy a boy and a girl a girl. Men have undergone a huge societal, relational and functional shift in the past 100 years. Some would say this has been detrimental and some progressive. One thing is certain: the identity of manhood, fatherhood and the male role in society has changed dramatically.

It is not possible to cover this subject exhaustively here but below are a few areas of consideration in men's health:

HEALTH TRENDS

1. Society

'Husbands love your wives, even as Christ also loved the church, and gave Himself for it.' **Ephesians 5:25**

Britain has the highest rate of marital breakdown in Europe. We live in a 'culture' of breakdown. There is a massive shift towards pre-marital sexual activity, cohabitation, extra-marital childbearing, divorce and decrease in marriage and fertility rates. In 1966 the UK had approximately 400,000 marriages compared to 310,000 in 1999. The age of first marriage has gone from 25 years for men in 1969 to 30 years in 1999.

Modern society is grappling for roles, expectations and responsibilities for men and women. There is a greater individualism and many of the more traditional concepts of relationships have been discarded. Modern man is often no longer the breadwinner, no longer the boss, no longer the parent and no longer the Prime Minister.

There is a great challenge today for men to identify the biblical model of manhood in its identity, its leadership and its function in the modern world. Many men are victims of modern society and need to find a personal wholeness in a strong identity in God the Father, brotherhood in Jesus Christ and function in the empowerment of the Holy Spirit. This will bring out the true image and likeness of God in men and their ministry.

There is a great challenge today for the church to raise godly leaders, spiritual fathers, male mentors and secure sons in the Christian faith. Our Christian heritage is full of pioneers, missionaries, reformers and revivalists. The church today often settles for great worship without great witness. It often focuses upon keeping the world out of the church instead of reaching the world with the church. Men benefit from a practical focus to their faith. Action men need to act and the church needs to connect with the modern man to release his potential.

There is a great challenge today for society to have positive male role models who make a difference to the world. Modern role models often come from the entertainment and sporting world. This can highlight some qualities of gifting and discipline but often focus on the fame and celebrity. Men of compassion, conviction and courage are needed to change the culture of our world.

2. Fathering

'For though you have ten thousand instructors in Christ, yet have ye not many fathers; for in Christ Jesus have I begotten you through the gospel.'

1 Corinthians 4:15

To have a child is easy, to raise a child is hard. All men have the potential to carry a son in their seed. Not all men raise the seed to become a son. We live in a fatherless generation and it is only now that we are beginning to understand the consequences of its legacy. If this generation is reaping the wind of fatherlessness, the next generation could reap the whirlwind. It is said that from the ages of 0-6 years old a mother is the strongest influence on a son's life. From 6-14 years it is the father and from 14 years onwards it is his peers. Fathers have a key role in shaping their sons identity and future.

Forty per cent of babies are now born outside of wedlock and 25 per cent of children are born to a single parent of which 98 per cent are women. Only one in 20 fathers receive custody of their children and a half of all divorced fathers only see their children once a week. Men are responsible for much of the above statistics but society has not wanted to acknowledge or accept the consequences that this is having on children.

80-90 per cent of juvenile criminals come from broken families and statistically without good role models boys naturally gravitate towards being bad ones. Children are clearly the victims of the modern world where individualism, secularisation and consumerism have eaten away at family values. Unfortunately these victims are now becoming tomorrow's parents and unless there is a radical change the future of men is a future of dysfunction. There is a hope. The church can be a voice of reform and restoration. God promises a spirit of adoption that can restore father-child relationships.

'Children are clearly the victims of the modern world. Unfortunately these victims are now becoming tomorrow's parents and unless there is a radical change the future of men is a future of dysfunction.'

And He shall turn the heart of the fathers to the children, and the heart of the children to the fathers, lest I come and smite the earth with a curse'.
Malachi 4:6

This is one of the most serious and important issues of the 21st century and is central to the ministry of the church. God is first a Father and has a Son (Jesus). Restoration of the father/child relationship is fundamental to salvation, wholeness and the well-being of a society.

3. Gender

'So God created man in His own image, in the image of God created He him, male and female created He them.' **Genesis 1:27**

The distinct separation of mankind in creation is male or female. Gender is not an issue of likeness; it is an issue of image. The image of God in creation reflects upon us maleness or femaleness as a fundamental conceptual identity. Image relates to what you reflect, likeness reflects what you do and how you behave. Homosexuality or same sex sexual relationships are issues of likeness and not image. The image is male or female but the likeness can reflect feelings, society, peers, emotions, thoughts, experiences, parenting, role modelling and influences. There are many reasons why homosexuality is so prevalent in our society today, but it is scripturally clear that God created a distinction in male or female.

Our image can be visually distorted in many ways:

1. Fatherlessness – absent fathers, passive fathers, and abusive fathers
2. Negative role models – figures of influence and authority in our lives who didn't fulfil their position of responsibility, e.g. teachers, ministers
3. Broken relationships – particularly abusive and dysfunctional ones

4. Societal trend – following the crowd
5. 'Spirit of the Age' – it is 'in the air' so people seem to catch it and follow it
6. Consumerism – desire to partake in every experience available
7. Environmental and nutritional – causing hormonal changes e.g. xeno-estrogens in plastics, which are thought to be affecting our hormonal equilibrium (this has not been proven yet)
8. Spiritual dispensation – many would say that there is a fundamental spiritual link to gender confusion related to the end times

All the above will not fundamentally change who we are in our created image but it could change how we see ourselves and what we become in this world. Ministry in this area requires a positive culture of personal healing and discipleship, strong positive role modelling of male-female relationships and leadership, growth in wholeness personally and relationally and practical lifestyle application.

4. Illicit and sexual behaviour

'Let no one despise your youth, but be an example to the believers in word, in conduct, in love, in spirit, in faith, in purity.' **1 Timothy 4:12**

The vast majority of paedophiles are men. 80 per cent of the victims of paedophilia are boys molested by adult males. It is estimated that 50 per cent of teenagers have tried illicit drugs. Long-term effects of the regular use of cannabis have yet to be proven but there is some evidence of its effect on motivation, educational attainment and long-term mental illness. Between 1996-2001 the rates of sexually transmitted disease increased significantly - Syphilis by 500 per cent, HIV by 256 per cent and Chlamydia by 108 per cent. The temptations and pressures in these areas are real. In a society where purity, chastity and abstinence are frowned upon it is all too easy for men to succumb to the environment around them in thought, word and deed.

A very real phenomenon that is drawing men in by the millions is 'net pornography'. The Daily Mail estimated that nearly 40 per cent of the adult male population logged onto sex websites in 2005. The UK is one of the most affected countries in the world with an overall porn industry worth an estimated £1 billion of the global £20 billion total. The sales of pornographic magazines have halved while the number of men downloading pornography has quadrupled in the past six years in the UK.

Why is this harmful?

1. It is against God's will. God created sex to be fulfilled within a monogamous relationship to one person of the opposite sex
2. It promotes covetousness, i.e. a desire for something that doesn't belong to you
3. It is self-seeking. It does not seek after the will of God. Lust seeks to satisfy itself; love seeks to satisfy God
4. It leads to retained and intrusive thoughts and memories that can impair peace, freedom and relationships
5. It leads to unrealistic expectations and comparisons of the present or future partner
6. It can give a derogatory perspective of the opposite sex that doesn't reflect the true image of God
7. It may lead to other forms of sexual gratification

How to be free?

1. Take it seriously. It can be pervasive and destructive
2. Seek genuine repentance and forgiveness
3. Don't overestimate your guilt and underestimate the sin
4. Find an accountability partner to openly, honestly and confidentially discuss your problem and progress with. Fully expose it to them so that deep healing can occur and chances of relapses are minimised

5. Identify trigger points for the behaviour, e.g. marital difficulties, singleness and set an action plan to resolve or manage them effectively
6. Place the highest level of filter on your P.C.
7. Only view the Internet in an open space
8. Install a programme that sends your weekly website hits to your accountability partner e.g.:
   www.cvmen.org.uk/resources.html
   www.covenanteyes.com
   www.xxxchurch.com

5. Psychological Well-being

'But we have the mind of Christ.' **1 Corinthians 2:16**

Suicide rates for men aged 15-24 have doubled between 1971 and 1999. Men are three times as likely to be murdered and four times as likely to commit suicide as women. Boys have a three times higher risk of Autism than girls.

The role of men in society and the home has changed dramatically and many men suffer from a crisis of confidence. This may show itself in passivity, timidity, lack of motivation and desire and even in sexual dysfunction. There is a gradual change of hormone levels with age in men but many suffer from real issues around identity, fulfilment and functional capacity.

There are at least 20 recognisable differences between the male and female brain. Men have fewer electrical connections between the right and left brain. The flow of information between the two is slower in the man. The speech centre is in the left and emotion centre in the right, hence it is harder and slower for a man to articulate emotions. The 'new man' seems more adept at this as society has encouraged him to be more expressive with his feelings and engage in social interactions at a more emotional level. It is true that many men have struggled with the demands and expectations of the modern man as society has changed in its structure and values.

It has been shown that men do their thinking in the more focussed regions of the brain. Men and women use the same part of the brain to handle emotions but women have stronger connections with this part of the brain and the language centre. Women tend to talk more about their problems and men tend to compartmentalise them and carry on unless they make a focussed conscious effort to talk about them.

Scriptural *Truth*

'For God has not given us the spirit of fear, but of power and of love and of a sound mind.' **2 Timothy 1:7**

'And the peace of God, which surpasses all understanding, will guard your hearts and mind through Christ Jesus.' **Philippians 4:7**

A sound and peaceful mind is a part of being healthy.

Several tips to a healthy mind:

- Know yourself – strengths and weaknesses, what drives you and moves you, vulnerability areas, likes and dislikes, generational and parental influences
- (Psalm 51:6)
- Be honest – it's the truth you know that makes you free (John 8:32)
- Learn to rest – faith and trust help you to 'switch off' from needs, demands and expectations (Hebrews 4:1-8)

'The role of men in society and the home has changed dramatically. Many men suffer from a crisis of confidence. This may show itself in passivity, timidity and even in sexual dysfunction.'

- Identify your love language – what makes you feel loved? For example being affirmed, physical touch, acts of service (e.g. a nice meal). If you are not receiving these things in your life from God or people you will feel undervalued, empty and alone (Luke 3:21-22)
- Avoid isolation – interaction, communication and relationships are a vital part of being healthy (Luke 8:27,38,39)
- Educate yourself – study, increase your knowledge, interests and learning (2 Timothy 2:15)
- Stimulate vision – do things that inspire, innovate and release creativity, spontaneity and purpose (Genesis 22:15-19)
- Reflect your ideas onto trusted friends as a safety net (Proverbs 24:6)
- Focus on the pure (Philippians 4:8)
- Avoid negative influences (2 Corinthians 10:4-5)
- Commit your thoughts to God (Philippians 4:6-7)

6. Physical well being

'And Moses was an hundred and twenty years old when he died: his eyes were not dim, nor his natural force abated'. **Deuteronomy 34:7**

Women live longer than men by an average of five years. The average of male death hasn't changed for a long time and is presently 75 years of age. There are several reasons for this including genetics and hormones but a large portion can be associated with high risk behaviour such as diet, exercise, alcohol, smoking, occupation etc. For men less than 75 years of age 40 per cent of deaths are due to heart disease and strokes and 30 percent cancer.
The number of males to females: at conception 120:100, at birth 105:100, at 35 100:100, at 60 80:100, at 80 60:100, at 100 12:100. Men start off in the majority and tail off dramatically after 35 years old.

Traditionally men have worse lifestyles, more risky occupations and rarely visit health care providers. Things are changing as we visit the 21st century women in the next chapter.

What kills men in the UK:

- Heart disease and stroke 40 per cent
- Cancers 32 percent – lung 10 per cent, prostate 4 per cent, colorectal 3 per cent, other 15 per cent
- Lung conditions excluding cancer e.g. asthma 9 per cent
- Injuries and poisoning 7 per cent
- All other causes 12 per cent

Positives

- Smoking is declining among men
- Men are more serious about health issues
- Men have bigger brains than women by 10 per cent but perform similarly intellectually – spare space for the ego!
- The government is recognising men's health as an issue with the first policy statement in 2002. Hopefully funding will follow

Negatives

- Death rates for young men aged 16-34 haven't significantly changed since 1971
- Suicide rates for young men aged 15-24 have doubled between 1971 and 1999
- The incidence of prostate and testicular cancer is increasing
- Erectile dysfunction is increasing – it is associated with heart disease, stress, and diabetes
- The number of men aged 25-64 dying from chronic liver disease has increased five-fold between 1970 and 2000, mostly related to alcohol misuse
- Hormone changes occur with age and some can affect energy, drive and motivation
- Male infertility appears to be on the increase and sperm quality and quantity reducing since the 1940's

- Recognition and funding for men's health issues have been neglected
- Rates of sexually transmitted infections have increased dramatically
- Obesity is higher in men and dramatically increases health risk

Take home points

- Take an interest – delay and denial can be a deadly cocktail
- Begin early – much of it is preventable with the right lifestyle
- Exercise regularly – bone thinning occurs with age
- No shame, you gain – check in with your doctor
- Know yourself – get to know your body to notice changes
- Never too late – you have to start somewhere, sometime. Why not now?
- Don't self destruct – have confidence in yourself before God
- Marriage is good, sex is healthy – research has shown that those who are married have more frequent and satisfying sexual relations. More frequent sex has been shown to improve the sense of smell, reduce the risk of heart disease, increase weight loss and overall fitness, reduce depression, improve pain relief, reduce colds and flu and give better bladder control. These apply to men and women. Indeed mortality risk was 50 per cent lower in the group with more frequent orgasms! God clearly made sex to be enjoyed and not endured

Summary

The issues of boyhood, fatherhood, brotherhood, maleness and manhood are often overlooked and neglected. Even within the bounds of Christian counselling and theology the link between the paternal side of God's nature, sonship and parenting are often confined to salvation and restoring the most basic of fathering relationships only. There is a fabric of life, relationships, society and church that is vitally linked to maleness and what it represents in its role and identity. We are only just beginning to realise the consequences of a society where these issues are sidelined and not addressed.

The celebration of a strong male identity from the cradle to the grave is complimentary to the awareness of femininity and female potential.
Jesus reflected true manhood from childhood to death. His life was respected, followed and received by men and women of all ages and backgrounds. His personal attention to His own spiritual, relational and physical life reflected in His ministry, mentoring and ultimately marriage to the church.

There is a great need for 21st century men to reflect the kind of manhood that Jesus represented on earth. Not only so that other men can be brought into wholeness and purpose but also to take their place in families, marriages and societies alongside women to see a restoration of godly homes and nations.

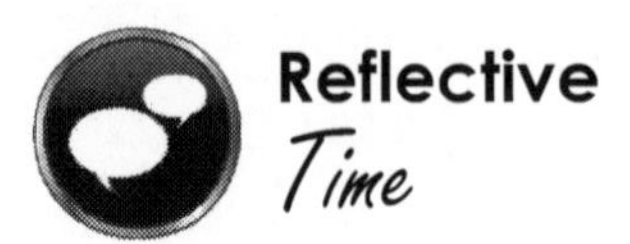

(30 minutes)

1. **What paternal influences have affected your life both positively and negatively?**
2. **What men do you respect and why?**
3. **What male biblical figure do you most admire and why?**

Personal *Thoughts*

CHAPTER SIXTEEN

WOMEN'S HEALTH

'And the rib, which the Lord God had taken from man, made He a woman, and brought her unto the man'. **Genesis 2:22**

1. Defining women

How do you define a woman? What is most important to her in a relationship with a man? What do women want? What fulfils women? Is it her nature to desire children? Can men understand women? Are women happy today? How much of a woman is nature and how much nurture?

These are all important questions for men, women and society. There is no doubt that a woman's role seems less clear than it used to be. They can be the major breadwinner, highest earner, lone parent, most spiritually aware, educationally successful and health conscious. Over the past 10 years however, women are beginning to suffer from traditionally male conditions of binge drinking, smoking, heart and liver disease as 21st century women cope with high levels of stress and multiple responsibilities.

Sex is a fixed issue of a biological male or female. Gender is how sexuality is affected by society, culture, upbringing and social structures. No two women are alike but the genetic predisposition of being a female is then impacted upon throughout a woman's life to define her femininity. Her desire for relationships, her ability to express emotion and communicate them with clarity, her appreciation for security and the attraction that comes from personal attention are all things that I suspect are common to most women. Most other facets of femininity and female personality may vary in intensity and importance among individual women.

2. What women want

In the film with Helen Hunt and Mel Gibson entitled 'What Women Want' the lead male character travelled an interesting journey trying to understand the make-up and needs of women. At the end of the film he asks the female character 'What do women want?' to which she replied 'they want to be understood but they want a man'. Many women think that men will never understand them and many men think it is impossible to understand women. How much difference this makes to the outcome of a relationship is difficult to know.

In a survey shown on the AOL home page in 2006 staff were asked what they thought members of the opposite sex wanted. Most men included flowers, gifts and security amongst their list of perceived women's wants. Many women listed sex as the No.1 male need from women. Overall, it seemed that being loved and accepted was the overriding desire and need of both sexes.

In a *Daily Mail* article (August 18th 2001 edition), it was noted that the actress Jane Fonda donated £9 million to a centre for gender and education saying 'money has been poured into making women strong in self belief but now its time to put the emphasis on boys to make them more like girls'. The shift in the educational success of women has been quite remarkable. In medicine there are two women to every one man entering medical school. In the 19th century women were considered too fragile for the profession.

3. Health trends

- **Historically**

1. *Health awareness* – there are more female-orientated magazines addressing health issues than male
2. *Health conscious* – women visit their doctor more frequently and are more proactive
3. *Health screening* – most cancer screening programmes relate to female

conditions such as breast and cervical cancer

4. *Health choices* – women tend to eat healthier and make healthier lifestyle choices than men
5. *Health responsibilities* – women often take the primary responsibility for health care within the family and make healthier choices, e.g. cease smoking when they become pregnant
6. *Health risks* – women have less risky occupations. Construction industry, etc is predominantly male
7. *Health relationships* – women express themselves more in the context of relationships and communicate more readily deeper issues of the soul–a problem shared is a problem halved
8. *Health spirituality* – women often lead in spiritual matters within the home and family such as prayer and church attendance
9. *Longevity* – women live on average five years longer than men. Is it any surprise looking at the above?

- **Presently (Things are changing)**

1. *Working patterns* – women are increasingly holding senior positions with positive and negative consequences and are often required to return to work after childbearing to maintain their lifestyle or meet financial needs
2. *Mental health* – stress is a major factor affecting the 21st century women juggling multiple tasks and roles. Recent evidence has also shown that there is a definite link between a previous abortion and long-term risk of adverse psychological consequences such as depression
3. *Family structure* – the explosion in single parenthood is the single most important determinant in health inequalities between rich and poor. Marriage is at an all time low and divorce at an all time high
4. *Risk behaviour* – binge drinking, antisocial behaviour, illicit drugs and sexual relationships are changing the profile of female illness and disease. Women are physically less able to detoxify alcohol at the same level as men. Sexually transmitted diseases such as Chlamydia, gonorrhoea, syphilis etc

have increased at alarming rates over the last decade

5. *Lifestyle* – obesity is of epidemic proportions within society as a whole but increasingly among women as they take on a sedentary unhealthy lifestyle. Smoking reduced from 1974 to 1994 but has increased since, particularly amongst the young
6. *Teenage pregnancy* – Britain has the highest rate in Europe. Availability of condoms and sex education in schools has failed to stop the rot
7. *Fertility* – women are marrying and having children later in life. Many factors affect fertility including nutrition, general well-being, mental state, weight and toxins but the largest factor is age. A women's fertility drops significantly as she ages and particularly after 30 years of age. Increasingly, women are turning to medical science to assist their fertility
8. *Relationships* – women are increasingly using the Internet for sexual purposes, though in different ways to men. They prefer to use chat rooms. Some women who enjoy frequent sex use cybersex as a way to engage in sexual activity in an uninhibited way. It is now such an industry that Anna Span, the UK's leading female porn director, makes films from a 'female point of view' with more 3-dimensional, foreplay and eye contact'! Singleness is an increasing problem for Christian women. A quarter of adult church attendees are single women while a tenth are men. Thirty per cent of the adult population generally remain single and 51 per cent of Londoners.
9. *Parenting* – over 6 million foetuses have been aborted since the abortion act of 1967

> *'Over 6 million foetuses have been aborted since the abortion act of 1967. In some quarters abortion is almost being promoted as a means of birth control.'*

In some quarters abortion is almost being promoted as a means of birth control. The woman often takes the consequences of the decision and carries the memories. Forty per cent of children are born outside of wedlock and single parents are largely women. Half of all divorced fathers see their children once a week so the burden of care is largely with the woman. Biblical guidelines to parenting are increasingly being sidelined in our secularising society.

10. *Self image* – it is estimated that up to a third of women have experienced some form of abuse (often sexual) in their lifetime. Forty per cent of young, homeless women experienced child abuse as a teenager. The effect of abuse is devastating and often leads to difficult or dysfunctional future relationships. Eating disorders are common in young women with occasional fatalities. Society's obsession with sex, body, media and entertainment creates huge pressures upon young women who feel compelled to conform to a perceived image

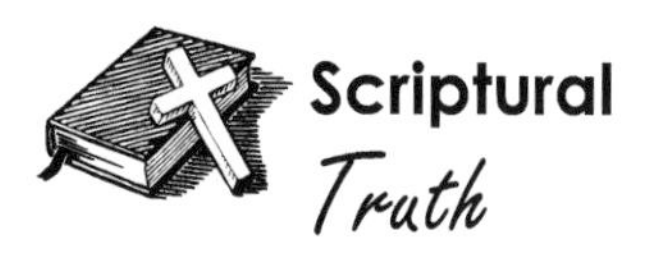

'I will praise You, for I am fearfully and wonderfully made; Marvellous are Your works, And that my soul knows very well.' **Psalm 139:14**

Future

What does the future hold for women? I am sure that most women would not want to return to bygone days. There is no doubt that women have undergone nothing short of a personal revolution in the past 100 years. In many ways their state has vastly improved in many parts of the world. In others they still suffer in silence with huge inequalities and limited rights. From cultural pressures in some societies to preferential boy births in others. From female circumcision to personal suicide on the death of her husband. Unfortunately, religion has often given God a bad name in this area.

In the bible God has expressed himself in maternal language and referred to wisdom and Jerusalem as its persona. Jesus spoke of wanting to gather the people of Jerusalem to Himself as a mother hen gathers her chicks. Jesus spoke personally, appropriately and respectfully to women. He empowered the woman at the well in John 4; he forgave the woman caught in adultery in John 8, and he healed the woman in rejection with the haemorrhage in Luke 8. He honoured his mother Mary in Luke 2:51 and was not afraid of godly intimacy with them in John 12:3. The woman was created in the image and likeness of God just as the man was (Genesis 1:26). There was no evidence of inequality in creation, only the need for one another (Genesis 2:18). It was a partnership with each holding specific strengths and qualities. They were made to fit.

One of the tragedies of the history of men and women has been the continual conflict and competition between them. This is a character of the fallen nature. Men need women and women need men to be complete. This is not just in the area of procreation, sexual fulfilment, marriage and family. To be healthy requires personal security in our masculinity and femininity as men and women but also the shared identity in reflecting God's image and likeness.

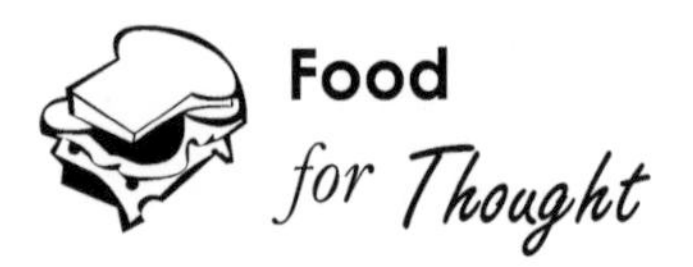

To be a whole person and whole society requires a return to the godly image of men and women reflecting the heart and hand of God in a unique and complementary way

Take home points

- In singleness–find contentment, look for character, cultivate friendship, stay accountable and trust God
- Body size isn't body image–don't self-destruct emotionally

God's image and God's likeness is to be who he made you to be

- Don't lose yourself in life–work, parenting and family can become your identity instead of reinforcing your identity
- Find a hobby
- Second best isn't God's best for you

'Charm is deceitful and beauty is passing, but a woman who fears the Lord, she SHALL be praised.' **Proverbs 31:30**

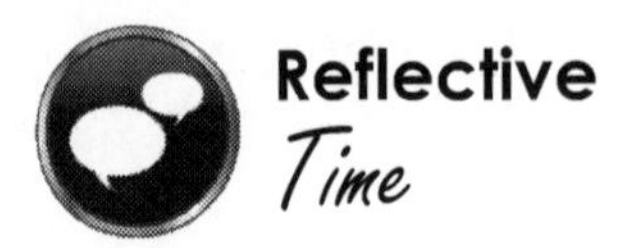

Reflective Time

(30 minutes)

1. **Which women have had the greatest impact upon your life?**
2. **What do you believe is God's vision for women and how does your life reflect that?**
3. **What female biblical figure do you most admire and why?**

Personal Thoughts

CHAPTER SEVENTEEN

AGEING

1. Introduction

This closing chapter could have been entitled youth, youthfulness, ageing or anti-ageing. I have chosen to call it ageing because that is what we all experience physically from the day we are conceived to the day we enter eternity. Death, however, is not the end but only a new beginning. We live in a society that wants to delay death at all costs and yet in other ways hasten death.

This is not the place for me to discuss euthanasia, physician-assisted suicide or abortion, as these issues require the proper attention and detail that is beyond the scope of this book. It is however true that the power of life and death are ultimately in God's realm. We can do much to alleviate suffering, delay death, enhance life and comfort loss but the gift of life belongs to God.

'Bless the Lord, O my soul and forget not all His benefits...Who satisfies your mouth with good things, so that your youth is renewed like the eagle's.'
Psalm 103:2,5

'For childhood and youth are vanity.' **Ecclesiastes 11:10**

'For me, to live is Christ, and to die is gain.' **Philippians 1:21**

'And as it is appointed unto men once to die, but after this the judgement'.
Hebrews 9:27

2. Purpose by design

The bible is very clear that the devil (thief) does not come except to steal, and to kill, and to destroy (John 10:10). In the beginning God created man in the garden to live forever without death, suffering or pain. This was and is the true heart of God towards us whatever we experience in this life and whatever happens in the world around us. God promises that for those who enter eternal paradise He 'will wipe away all tears from their eyes; and there shall be no more death, neither sorrow, nor crying, neither shall there be any more pain; for the former things are passed away' (Revelation 21:4). Death will ultimately be cast into the lake of fire (Revelation 20:14).

In the beginning and the end God is for life. The Garden of Eden had a tree of life and a tree of knowledge of good and evil. Man chose the tree of knowledge and he lost life physically, spiritually and interpersonally with himself and others. Knowledge is not wrong but to choose knowledge above life is seeking to elevate man above creature into creator. Nowhere is this truer than in the knowledge of good and evil. Throughout history there have been people who thought they were doing what was good but in fact were destroying many lives.

3. Morality and life as the realm of God

Good, evil, morality and ethics are often influenced by the age in which we live, the vocal minorities and the opinions of the majorities. Defining good and evil is in the realms of God and if we seek to govern humanly then we elevate ourselves beyond ourselves. Heaven will have no tree of knowledge, only a tree of life (Revelation 22:1-5). If there was any doubt to God being pro-life then it was demonstrated further through His son.

Jesus brought forgiveness, hope, peace, healing, deliverance, restoration and reconciliation as He went about 'doing good' (Acts 10:38). In contrast to Satan the scripture I alluded to earlier clearly demarcates the difference in purpose. Jesus said 'I am come that they might have life, and that they might have it more abundantly.' (John 10:10).

4. Palliative Care

Palliative care is a field of medicine that was set up to alleviate the suffering of the dying, prepare for death and caring for the terminally ill. They are increasingly recognising the importance of the spiritual needs of patients in their integrated practice. Originally focussing upon cancer patients they are now extending their services to others with terminal illness.

5. Issues of ageing

In looking at biblical health and ageing it would be easy to focus just on longevity of life. Longevity must have a context and a purpose and hence viewing ageing from a total perspective is very important to give this purpose and context. Life without meaning gives no meaning to life. Ageing without eternity gives no continuity of purpose.

Society today promotes youth (through the race and pace of 21st century life and living), preserves youthfulness (through self help and self development), prevents ageism (through laws and policies) and prolongs anti ageing (through lifestyle and prosperity). In contrast, however, it prevents youth (through despising innocence, experiencing 'the world', educational values), shortens youthfulness (through family and societal breakdown), promotes ageism (undervalues experience, despises authority, idolises individuality) and reduces anti-ageing (through health inequalities).

Life without meaning gives no meaning to life. Ageing without eternity gives no continuity of purpose.

These conflicting parallels highlight the deeper issues around age and ageing. The first four scriptures in this chapter draw to our attention four issues of ageing:

- **The blessing of youth - longevity**
- **The vanity of youth - youthfulness**
- **The purpose of youth - productivity**
- **The process of youth - eternity**

The blessing of youth - longevity

Age is a taboo subject. I am sure we all know people who will defend to the grave anyone finding out their age. This can be cultural, as within certain countries and cultures people may not speak about their age. It may be personal, as there can be experiences or superstitions around age. Or it may be a gender issue. Generally women are more reluctant to divulge their age than men though I have definitely met men who are quite tetchy about revealing their age!

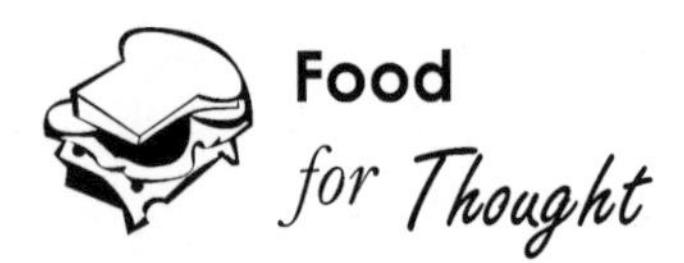

People say that getting old is all in the mind. This is true but it is also in the body. It is not so much whether you get old that is in the mind as this is guaranteed, but how you get old is in the mind. Rigor mortis will set in when you die but don't let it set into your thinking before you die!

We are an ageing population. Twelve million people (20 per cent of the population) are over 60 years old in the UK at present and it is projected to rise to 18.6 million (30 per cent of the population) by 2031. Some would say that we are more ageist and some would say that we are living longer 'iller'.

There is no doubt that quantity of life isn't always quality of life. Social isolation, family breakdown, community disrespect and changing values have undermined many of the pivotal roles of older people in our society. Malnutrition among the elderly is widespread. It is estimated that one in seven older adults are at risk of under nutrition and those in institutions such as nursing homes being the most at risk. The average life expectancy for men is 74-75 years of age and for women 79-80 years of age. It is estimated that by 2030 there will be more older people in the USA than younger people. These are huge concerns for politicians and health economists as they try to weigh up the financial implications of an ageing population.

Biblical longevity

After the flood at the time of Noah, God limited man's lifespan to 120 years (Genesis 6:3). It is interesting to note that it is exceedingly rare in recorded history other than in scriptural text for anyone to live beyond 120 years. The oldest recorded people tend to live to 110-115 maximum. Prior to Noah's time it was not unusual for people to live several hundred years, even after the Fall in the Garden of Eden.

Many people find this hard to believe but it is presumptuous to assume that we can judge previous generations solely on the basis of present knowledge since no living person was around 5000 years ago. Archaeological evidence is changing our understanding of history and there are many archaeological findings, which are confirming some of the ancient biblical events. Some modern anti-ageing therapists believe that it is possible for every human to live to 120 years in the right environment and lifestyle.

An article in *Time* magazine made an in interesting observation in looking at cells in the human body. Our cells are programmed to live and survive. Ageing results from a gradual accumulation of faults in the cells and tissues. There are no death genes and cell death is the body's way of getting rid of damaged cells. Our genes account for 25 per cent of what determines length of life by regulating repair and maintenance. Seventy-five per cent of what determines length of life is determined by individual variability based on nutrition, lifestyle, exercise and environment. This determines our exposure to damage and capacity to repair. It may well be true then what the Chinese proverb says: *'Until you are 40 you have the face you are born with. After 40 you have the face you deserve'.*

A survey of older people once asked 'What would you do if you had your life over again?' They said rest more, reflect more and risk more.

The vanity of youth – youthfulness

You can't stop the rot but you may be able to delay it. Youthfulness means to be youth-full, i.e. full of youth – in thinking, in body, in belief, in vision and in purpose.

Women live on average five years longer than men. It was thought that this was mainly genetic in nature but it would appear that many other factors contribute to this. For example cancer screening has been largely focussed on women over the past 25 years. Women are more proactive and health aware, women's health as a medical field has been far more advanced and developed than men's health and women have historically had less lifestyle risk factors such as smoking, alcohol, diet and occupation.

On studying centenarian populations in the world, which have the highest number of people who live to 100 years old, certain critical factors have contributed to their state. Not smoking, not excessive amounts of alcohol, a Mediterranean-type diet, being part of a community, marriage, having a faith and a strong family unit where older members still play an active part.

One other factor, which came out of a study in America on longevity, was that the presence of a pioneering spirit defined as an interest in new things and an enthusiasm for change was at the root of longevity. It is also true to say that many of the above apply to longevity of life generally but centenarians do also have a stronger genetic component.

Psalm 90:10 says 'The days of our years are threescore years and ten (70 years); and if, by reason of strength, they be fourscore years (80)...'
The word strength denotes 'might'. This can be used in the context of God's strength in us but also our effort 'with all one's might'.

Much of what can make a difference to quality **AND** quantity of life I have alluded to earlier. There is, however, a partnership between what God can do FOR us (grace), IN us (healing) and THROUGH us (vision) and what we can do for ourselves (personal responsibility in health, home, church and life), in ourselves (trust, letting go, forgiveness, yieldedness) and through ourselves (hard work, diligence, faithfulness). Understanding this partnership and outworking it in our lives is critical in doing all that we can do to fulfil God's desire and plan for our lives. There are two ways of viewing the process of the ages we pass through in life:

The Shakespearean model

All the world's a stage and the men and women mere players; they have their exits and entrances. And one man in his time plays many parts. His acts being seven ages.

- Infancy
- Whining schoolboy (childhood)
- Lover (adolescent)
- Soldier (young adult)
- Justice (adult)
- Retirement (old age)
- Second childishness and mere oblivion (dementia and death)

(Poem Lyrics of Seven Ages of Men by William Shakespeare)

These seven stages seem to be comments on human development by William Shakespeare. People interpret them in different ways including some associating them with the carnal nature of the seven deadly sins of wrath, greed, lust, envy, gluttony, sloth and pride.

I am sure not all Shakespearean connoisseurs will agree but there have been many attempts to look at the human life through the ages. There is no offence meant in using William Shakespeare as an example of a human development model.

The Biblical model

While man fears change, God embraces change and the progression of human life from dependant child to independent teenager to interdependent adult is a progress of growth and development. Each stage has its advantages and disadvantages but the important point is not the pros and cons of each stage of our life but what God is trying to teach us through each stage and His purpose in that. Failure to understand the purpose and the process will lead to lost time, a life of regret and a longing for 'the good old days'. Many people have life crisis associated with age and while it is not possible to turn back the clock it is possible to redeem the time. Though we live forever, we live now only once. We can learn from the past, live for the present and look to the future.

Here are my thoughts on the seven ages of man:

- Infancy – Dependence and hunger
- Childhood – Innocence and purity
- Adolescence – Learning and exploring
- Young adult – Energy, vision and vitality
- Adult – Maturity
- Old age – Wisdom and reflection
- Deathbed – Legacy

There are spiritual principles that can be learnt from each stage and added to by the following stage. Growing older isn't always moving on. We can still appreciate and learn from those who are coming through subsequent stages and generations. It is not crisis management but growth management and understanding these principles can help us find purpose, whatever our stage in life.

Grey hairs are not the first sign of rigor mortis but of life experience. Wrinkles are lifelines and not death lines.

Tests (from God), trials (from the world) and temptations (from Satan) can change with age. The seven deadly sins are deadly. We can be cut down in the flower of any age and it is important to know that a lifetime of building can be brought down by a moment of madness. Each stage can only profit from the previous stage if maintained in humility and purity. God can restore, revive and renew but prevention is better than cure. Restoring what's lost would not be necessary if we didn't lose it in the first place. Take time to nurture and care for what you have so you don't waste time trying to get back what you've lost.

There is a pointlessness to youth as mentioned in Ecclesiastes 11:10 because it cannot be an end in itself. Eternal youth is not a physical reality but it can be a spiritual reality based on our attitude, belief, mindset and lifestyle. The point to youth is its purpose in the whole. In finding that purpose you can enjoy your youth to the full and be renewed in your youth daily.

The diagram below shows what happens often in our lives with age as we grow beset by the cares, disappointments and responsibilities of life and a sense of worldliness begins to creep in.

God/Spirit	Self/Soul	World/Body	Godliness
God/Spirit	World/Body	Self/Soul	Carnality
Self/Soul	God/Spirit	World/Body	Soulish
Self/Soul	World/Body	God/Spirit	Selfishness
World/Body	Self/Soul	God/Spirit	Worldliness

The progression is from a godly (spirit first) life through to a worldly focussed life. This transition does not happen quickly and it can be a slow regression over many years in response to unwise choices, pressures, circumstances and disappointments. It can happen at any age but the tragedy is that it often robs us of the very life we desire.

'He gives power to the weak; and to those who have no might He increases strength. Even the youths shall faint and be weary, and the young men shall utterly fall, but those who wait on the Lord shall renew their strength; they shall mount up with wings like eagles, they shall run and not be weary, They shall walk and not faint.' **Isaiah 40:29-31**

If your body fails you, keep your mind; if your mind fails you, keep your spirit; and if your spirit fails you, its time to go home!

The purpose of youth – productivity

In looking at the effectiveness of our life it is important to understand three phrases:

1. *God's Providence* – His ability to see what we cannot see and to know what we do not know and to make things happen in such a way as to do what He has planned to do
2. *God's Plan* – His set design in fulfilling his will
3. *God's Purpose* – His goal

With age there should be productivity to our life. God's first commandment to Adam and Eve was one of a productive life. *'Then God blessed them, and God said to them, "Be fruitful, and multiply, and fill the earth, and subdue it; and have dominion...".'* **Genesis 1:28**

Fruit is first rooted in the seed, sprouted in the stem, grows through the plant and fruits from the branch. This is a process that occurs with time and requires the right food and climate. In an ideal setting we would meet our maker in childhood, find a mission in youth, mature in adulthood and multiply in parenthood and grandparenthood. A life like this will leave a legacy.

Our life should not be just a series of experiences but a continual journey of purpose in God through the years.

There are many facets of productivity but a clear sense of providence, plan and purpose will help us to keep perspective and keep progressing towards our God given goal. Providence is to know that God knew you before you knew you; He was working behind the scene to create the scene. He is the bigger picture. God has a definite and distinct plan for our lives that is crafted into our spiritual DNA. As we walk 'the way' then we learn the will. In the providence is a plan and in the plan there is a purpose. Purpose is not merely what you do, it is who you are.

You are part of an eternal story that is being played out all around you. We are not the end in itself. God has a part for us to play but we are not the centre stage. We live for today but we are part of tomorrow. Our life in our lifetime is significant in determining whether Christ's kingdom will be extended. Trusting God's providence, finding His plan and fulfilling His purpose is central to a fruitful life.

The process of youth – eternity

Being aware of your own mortality can be a good thing. Recognising that you are not the architect and controller of every aspect of your life can be very releasing. Knowing God - who is omnipresent, omniscient and omnipotent - can help you find hope, faith, peace and rest within yourself and with others.

Most people don't want to ask the ultimate question of 'where will I go when I die?' because they either don't know the answer or don't want to know the answer. They then settle for the path of least resistance which evolutionary theory can provide. Many people would disagree with this but I find a huge amount of presumption, assumption and theory within evolution that defies a scientific rational mind. Most people live on earth between 60 to 80 years. Their philosophy of youth is often 'eat, drink and be merry for tomorrow we may die'.

People spend years researching medicine at University, hours researching finances in the latest mobile phones and a lifetime researching relationships in marriage. They often spend no time researching God in their heart.
If you are a risk taker you could choose to believe in God and probably have nothing to lose. You could also choose not to believe in God and have everything to lose. If you are a risk manager you could at least research the options until you find rest in your soul and then make a choice. Most people rely on others to make this choice for them and risk everything.
One thing is for certain. The bible says that there is an eternity. There is one life on earth and one judgement in eternity. There is no reincarnation or reinvention. If that is true then we have one life to get it right. If eternity is forever then we will forever live with the choice we make.

It is also true that because many people have not found rest within their soul on the issue of death and eternity their quality and quantity of life is affected on earth. Would every suicide take place if everyone knew what came next? Having eternal security can help you put circumstances, relationships, ambitions and needs in context, which can give you greater peace and rest in dealing with daily life on earth.

Some deep issues of rejection, fear and shame can also find a haven in knowing that an eternal God knows, watches and cares about your life.

It will help you resolve issues of justice and righteousness in a world that is often unfair and unjust. Seeing the bigger picture is very important in bringing biblical health to a logical and truthful conclusion. I hope you have enjoyed and will fulfil the journey.

Summary

- Live spirit first, soul second, body third. The spiritual is eternal, the physical is temporal and the soul is interrelation. Eternal principles have temporal effects that bring a quality and quantity to life
- Be a risk taker and not just a risk manager
- Resist wrong, rest well, reflect much and risk a lot
- Little changes over a long time are better than large changes over a short time
- What you sustain, you maintain and gain
- Let your life leave a legacy and your home a heritage
- Live forever in Christ but live NOW
- Learn from the past, live for the present, look to the future
- Trust providence, find a plan and fulfil purpose

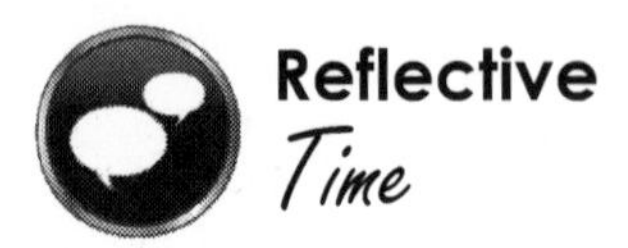

(20 minutes)

1. **Have you answered the ultimate question - 'where will I spend eternity?'**
2. **Looking back on your life, what can you change to make a better future?**
3. **How can you make your life more fruitful?**
4. **What can you do today to improve your quality and longevity of life?**

Personal Thoughts

CONCLUSION

In preparing this book I have been conscious of the fact that the subject covered is so vast as to cover our whole lives and all it represents. Health is more than physical and incorporates our total relational world and spiritual being.

The Old English language was derived from the Germanic, Anglo-Saxon language. In this ancient derivation comes the meaning of the word health. The word has one root, which is the same for body and soul – hal. This word 'health' coming from that root, means 'health', 'whole' and 'holy'. These three meanings were used interchangeably and clearly show that 'to be healthy' means 'to be whole' which means 'to be holy'. The physical expression in its ideal would represent physical and mental performance, absence of ill health and longevity. Biblically, it is clear that God created marriage, family, community and the church. The nations are held together by these core relational entities and fulfilling relationships are vital to our sense of belonging and identity.

Our central anchor in health, however, is none of the above and is the most neglected aspect of global health today. Billions of pounds are spent tackling global health issues but the most important solution is available to all at no financial cost.

Jesus made a statement which still shakes the world today:

'I am the way, the truth and the life: no man cometh unto the Father, but by me.' **John 14:6**

The health industry is often a confused sound of conflicting opinions and agendas. Nowhere is this more evident than in the area of spiritual health. Reiki, Transcendental meditation, pilgrimages, psychology in the paranormal and crystal healing all seek to link the human personality to a spiritual dimension. Jesus makes a definitive statement that cancels out all other claims in this area.

He claims to be THE way, THE truth and THE life. The reason for this is very simple. Spirituality is not a force or a supreme being, it is a person. God is a Spirit but God is also a Father. When man lost relationship with God as a result of sin he lost the essence of who he was. Jesus was the God-man, man-God who died to restore that relationship through His death on the cross and resurrection from the dead. He took our sin that we might be forgiven. That is the only WAY to spiritual health, it is the only TRUTH that has evidence and experience to back it up and it is the only LIFE that will take us from temporal health in this world to eternal health in the next.

If you find a greater vitality and wellness as a result of this book I will be pleased.
If your marriage is improved, your family enhanced and your community more involved as a result of this book I will be delighted.
If your life is empowered, your future envisioned and your ministry enlivened as a result of this book I will be overjoyed.
But if you find Christ as a result of this book, then its purpose will have been fulfilled.

'For God so loved the world, that he gave His only begotten Son, that whoever believes in Him should not perish, but have everlasting life.' **John 3:16**

REFERENCES

All scriptural quotations — King James/New King James Version Bible. All concordance references — 'Young's Analytical Concordance To The Bible' (ISBN 0-8407-4945-7).

All word definitions — 'Compact Oxford English Dictionary' Third Edition (ISBN 0-19-861428-4).

CHAPTER 1 — BIBLICAL BASIS

Any references are stated in the chapter

CHAPTER 2 — PURPOSE

- Brignall, I. (2003) 'You matter to the last moment of your life', *British Medical Journal*, 12 June 2003, Vol. 326, p 1335

CHAPTER 3 — THE MIND

- Dorling, D., S. Frankel, D. Gunnell, N. Middleton & E. Whitley (2002), 'Why are suicide rates rising in young men but falling in the elderly?', *Social Science & Medicine,* Vol. 57 No. 4, August 2003 , pp. 595-611
- Harris, S. (2002) *Marriage 'will be extinct in 30 years',* Internet www page at URL: http://lists101.his.com/pipermail/smartmarriages/2002-April/001096.html
- Smart Marriages (2002) *Tackle juvenile crime 'by strengthening marriage',* Internet www page at URL: http://lists101.his.com/pipermail/smartmarriages/2002-April/001096.html
- BBC NEWS (2006) *Births out of wedlock 'pass 40%'* , Internet www page at URL: http://news.bbc.co.uk/1/hi/uk/4733330.stm
- UK Men and Father's Rights, '6. Statistics', Internet www page at URL: http://www.coeffic.demon.co.uk/stats.htm
- National Statistics (2005), 'Focus on families 2004' Internet www pages at URL:http://www.statistics.gov.uk/downloads/theme_compendia/fof2005/

families.pdf

CHAPTER 4 — THE EMOTIONS

- Chapman, G (1995) *The Five Love Languages,* U.S.: Northfield Publishing

CHAPTER 5 — THE WILL

Any references are stated in the chapter

CHAPTER 6 — FOOD

- Holford, P. (1997) *The Optimum Nutrition Bible,* London: Piatkus Books
- Atkins, R.C. (1999) *Dr Atkins New Diet Revolution*, London: Vermilion
- Brand-Miller, J., S. Colagiuri, K. Foster-Powell & A. Leeds, (1998) *The GI Factor,* London: Coronet Books
- Baur, L., E.J. Elliot & D.E Thomas (2007) 'Low glycemic index or low glycemic load diets for overweight and obesity', *Cochrane database of systemic reviews 2007*, issue 3
- Gandini, S., P. Gnagnarella, C. La Vecchia & P. Maisonneuve (2008) 'Glycemic index, glycemic load, and cancer risk: a meta-analysis' *American Journal of Clinical Nutrition*, June 2008, Vol. 87, pp 1793 - 1801
- Liu, S., J. Manson & W. Willett (2002), 'Glycemic index, glycemic load, and risk of type 2 diabetes[1,2,3]', *The American Journal of Clinical Nutrition*, July 2002, Vol. 76 No. 1, pp 274 - 280

CHAPTER 7 — WATER

- United Nations Department of Information (2002) *Johannesburg Summit Secretary-General calls for global action on water issues*, Internet www pages at URL:http://www.un.org/jsummit/html/media_info/pressrelease_prep2/global_action_water_2103.pdf
- Wikimedia Foundation Inc. (2008) *Purified water*, Internet www page at URL:http://en.wikipedia.org/wiki/Distilled_water
- Wikimedia Foundation Inc.(2008) *Reverse osmosis*, Internet www page at URL:http://en.wikipedia.org/wiki/Reverse_osmosis

- Heartspring (2008), *Clinical studies on the effects of electrolyzed-reduced water-ionized water*, Internet www page at URL:http:/ www.heartspring.net/water_clinical_studies.html
- Whitfield, H.N. (2006) 'Too much of a good thing?', *British Journal of General Practice*, volume 56, pp 542-544
- Scrivner, J. (2002) 'Water, water everywhere!', *The Star*, pp 14
- Peden, J. (2002) 'Is bottled water better than normal tap water?', *Pulse*, volume 62, number 4, pp 112

CHAPTER 8 — SLEEP

- Cappuccio, F. (2006) 'Sleep deprivation increases obesity risk', *Update*, August 2006, pp7, 9
- Hart-Davis, A. (2005) 'A genius pill: would you really be stupid to swallow it?, *The Scotsman*, December 2nd 2005
- Gorman, C. (2005) 'Why we sleep', *Time*, 24 January, pp 40-50
- Britton, T., N. Douglas, A. Hansen, J. Hicks, R. Howard, A. Meredith, I. Smith, G. Stores, S. Wilson, Z. Zaiwalla & A. Zeman (2004) 'Narcolepsy and excessive daytime sleepiness', *British Medical Journal*, 25 September 2004, Vol. 329, pp 724-728
- Wynne-Jones, M. (2003) 'Advising a poor sleeper on Melatonin', *Pulse*, June 2003, pp 66-68
- Watkins, S. (2000) 'Poverty of sleep-debt society', *Health and Aging*, January 2000, pp 36
- D'Agostino, R.B., M. D. Lebowitz, B. K. Lind, A. B. Newman, F. J. Nieto, T. G. Pickering, S. Redline, J. M. Samet, E. Shahar & T. B. Young (2000) 'Association of Sleep-Disordered Breathing, Sleep Apnea, and Hypertension in a Large Community-Based Study', *The Journal of the American Medical Association*, 12 April 2000, Vol. 284 No. 14, pp 1829-1836
- Babineau, T.W, B. P. Eng, H. R. Feldman, R. D. Vorona, J. C. Ware, M. P. Winn (2005) 'Overweight and Obese Patients in a Primary Care Population Report Less Sleep Than Patients With a Normal Body Mass Index', *Archives*

of Internal Medicine, 10 January 2005, Vol. 165 No. 1, pp 25-30

- Cauter, E.V., R. Leproult & K. Spiegel (1999) 'Impact of sleep debt on metabolic and endocrine function', *Lancet*, 23 October 1999, Vol. 354, Issue 9188, pp 1435-1439
- Adams, J. (2006) 'Socioeconomic position and sleep quantity in UK adults', *Journal of Epidemiology and Community Health* , Vol. 60, pp 267-269
- Johns, M.W (1991) 'A New Method For Measuring Daytime Sleepiness: The Epworth Sleepiness Scale ', *Sleep*, Vol. 14 No.6, pp 540-545

CHAPTER 9 — LAUGHTER

- Adams, P. (2000) 'Laughter: the best medicine', *WDDTY*, February 2000, pp 12
- Coghlan, A. (2005) 'Laughing helps arteries and boosts blood flow', New Scientist, 12 March 2005, Issue 2490
- Cousins, N. (1989) Head first: *The biology of hope,* New York: Dutton
- Layard, R, (2005) *Happiness: Lessons from a new science*, U.S.A.: Penguin Publishing

CHAPTER 10 — EXERCISE

- Abrams, K.R., N.J. Cooper, C.L. Gillies, R.T. Hsu, K. Khunti, P.C. Lambert & A.J. Sutton (2007) 'Pharmacological and lifestyle interventions to prevent or delay type 2 diabetes in people with impaired glucose tolerance: systematic review and meta-analysis', *BMJ*, 10 February 2007, Vol. 334, pp 299-302
- Morris, J.N. (1994) 'Exercise in the prevention of coronary heart disease: today's best buy in public health', *Medicine & Science in Sports & Exercise*, July 1994, Vol. 26(7), pp 807-814
- Ashton, W.D., K. Nanchahal & D.A. Wood (2000) 'Leisure-time physical activity and coronary risk factors in women', *Journal of Cardiovascular risk*, August 2000, Vol. 7(4), pp 259-266
- Appel, L.J., L. Belden, C. Bragg, A. Brewer, J. Cohen, N.R. Cook, I. Lee, M. Mattfeldt-Beman, N.C. Milas, M. Millstone, J. Raczynski, B. Singh, V.J.

Stevens, E. Obarzanek & D.S. West (2001) 'Long-Term Weight Loss and Changes in Blood Pressure: Results of the Trials of Hypertension Prevention, Phase II', Annals of Internal Medicine, January 2001, Vol. 134 Issue 1, pp 1-11

- Levi, F., F. Lucchini, C. Pasche, A. Tavani, C. La Vecchia (1999) 'Occupational and leisure-time physical activity and the risk of colorectal cancer', *European Journal of Cancer Prevention*, December 1999, Vol. 8(6), pp 487-494
- Colditz, G. A., S. E. Hankinson, D.J. Hunter, J.E. Manson, B. Rockhill, W.C. Willet (1999) 'A Prospective Study of Recreational Physical Activity and Breast Cancer Risk', Archives in Internal Medicine, 25 October 1999, Vol. 159, No. 19, pp 2369-2370
- Johnson, M.J., A.W Taylor (2007) *Physiology of exercise and healthy aging*, Human Kinetics Publishers

CHAPTER 11 — FASTING

- Bueno-Aguer, L. (1991) *Fast your way to health*, U.S.: Whitaker House
- Braverman, E. (1994) 'The benefits of fasting', *Total Health*, June 1994, Vol. 16 Issue 3

  Anderson, S.V., T.C. Campbell, A. Goldhamer, D. Lisle & B. Parpia (2001) 'Medically supervised water-only fasting in the treatment of hypertension', *Journal of Manipulative and Physiological Therapeutics* , Vol. 24 Issue 5, pp 335-339
- National Institute on Aging, U.S. National Institutes of Health (2003) *Meal skipping helps rodents resist Diabetes, brain damage,* Internet www page at URL:http://www.nia.nih.gov/NewsAndEvents/PressReleases/PR20030428MealSkipping.htm
- National Institute on Aging, U.S. National Institutes of Health (2003) *Fasting forestalls Huntington's Disease in mice*, Internet www page at URL:http://www.nia.nih.gov/NewsAndEvents/PressReleases/PR20030210Fasting.htm
- Carroll, W. (2002) *The health benefits of fasting*, Internet www page at

URL:http://serendip.brynmawr.edu/exchange/node/1834

- Stephensen, C.B (2001) 'Examining the effect of a nutrition intervention on immune function in healthy humans: what do we mean by immune function and who is really healthy anyway?', *American Journal of Clinical Nutrition,* November 2001, Vol. 74 No. 5, pp 565-566
- Jolly, C. A. (2004) 'Dietary restrictions and immune function', *The American Society for Nutritional Sciences,* August 2004, Vol. 134, pp 1853-1856
- Heilbronn, L.K, E. Ravussin & J.V. Smith (2004) 'Energy restriction and aging' *Current Opinion in Clinical Nutrition & Metabolic Care,* November 2004, Vol. 7, pp 612-622
- Shimokawa, I. & Y. Higami (2001) 'Leptin & anti-aging action of caloric restriction', *The Journal of nutrition, health & aging,* 2001, Vol. 5 No.1, pp 43-48
- Atkinson, R. L., A. Bartke, G.A. Bray, J.N. Crawley, C.E. Finch, E. Maratos-Flier, C.V. Mobbs & J.F. Nelson (2001) 'Neuroendocrine and Pharmacological Manipulations to Assess How Caloric Restriction Increases Life Span', *The Journals of Gerontology Series A: Biological Sciences and Medical Sciences* , 2001, Vol. 56, pp 34-44
- Ehret, A. (1966) *Rational fasting for physical, mental and spiritual rejuvenation,* New York: Ehret Literature Publishing Co.

CHAPTER 12 — NUTRITION

The optimum nutrition Bible, Patrick Holford – see above

CHAPTER 13 — REST

Any references are stated in the chapter (excluding BBC International Monetary Fund)

CHAPTER 14 — STRESS

- Pinker, S. (2007) 'The mystery of consciousness', *Time,* February 12th 2007, pp 41-61

- Womack, S. (2007) *'Stressful days at work "turn one in three to drink',* Internet www page at URL:http://www.telegraph.co.uk/news/uknews/1541238/Stressful-days-at-work-%27turn-one-in-three-to-drink%27.html
- Morgan, C. (2007) 'The stress slayers', *Higher Nature*, 2007, pp 10
- Cooper, C. (2006) 'Fifteen minutes with... An occupational psychologist and anti-stress sage', *BMJ Careers*, December 9th 2006, pp 215-218
- Theorell, T. & R.A. Karasek (1996) 'Current issues relating to psychosocial job strain and cardiovascular disease research', *Journal of Occupational Health Psychology*, January 1996, Vol. 1, pp 9-26
- Anderson, D.R., R.Z. Goetzel, R.J. Ozminkowski, S. Serxner, J. Wasserman, R. W. Whitmer & Health Enhancement Research Organization HERO Research Committee (2000) 'The Relationship Between Modifiable Health Risks and Group-level Health Care Expenditures', *American Journal of Health Promotion,* September 2000, Vol. 15 Issue 1, pp 45-52

CHAPTER 15 — MEN'S HEALTH

- Gould, D. D. (2007) 'Managing the andropause', *Update,* January 2007, pp 63-68
- Ripley, A. (2005) 'Who says a woman can't be Einstein', *Time*, March 7th 2005, pp 52-56
- Black, D. (2006) 'Caring for the elderly male', *Geriatric Medicine*, September 2006, pp 5-25
- Ford, C. & U. Gordon (2004) 'Why male fertility is about more than just sperm count', *Pulse*, January 26th 2004, pp 49-52
- Bartholomew, R (YEAR?) 'Natural and effective support for male sexual function and vitality', *Nutri News,* issue no. 97
- Petter, K. (YEAR?) 'Nutrition support for prostatic health', *Nutri News*, issue no. 60
- Schering Health Care (2006), 'Male Hypogonadism', *Pulse Quick Guides*, July 2006

- Delvin, D. (2001) 'Lack of libido in men', *Doctor*, April 2001, pp 84-88
- Charlton, R. & G. Smith (2002), 'Key facts on problems of men's health', *Pulse*, February 25th 2002, pp 80
- Imm, N. (2002) 'Men's health is no better 30 years on', *Pulse*, June 10th 2002, pp 56
- Wood, S. (2000) 'A guide to common conditions of the penis', *The Practitioner*, September 2000, pp 728-736
- Daily Mail (2006), Downloads of porn hit record high, *Daily Mail*, 29 May 2006
- Lott, T. (2006) 'I look at porn, am I a monster?', *The Independent*, 28 May 2006
- Barnes, A. & S Goodchild (2006) 'Porn UK', *The Independent*, 28 May 2006
- Shalit, W. (1999) *A return to modesty: discovering the lost virtue'*, Free Press

CHAPTER 16 — WOMEN'S HEALTH

- Kemm, J. R. (2001) 'A birth cohort analysis of smoking by adults in Great Britain 1974 - 1998', *Journal of Public Health Medicine*, December 2001 volume 23, issue 4, pp 306 - 311
- Babb, P & J. Matheson (2002) 'Social Trends', *National Statistics*, No. 32, 2002 edition
- Freely, M. (2002) 'What children really think about divorce', *The Guardian*, 24 January 2002
- Office for National Statistics (2001) Census 2001
- Cooper, C.L. & V.J. Sutherland (1993) 'Identifying distress among general practitioners : predictors of psychological ill-health and job dissatisfaction', *Social science and medicine*, 1993, Vol. 37, No. 5, pp 575-581
- Gardiner, M. & M. Tiggermann (1999) 'Gender differences in leadership style, job stress and mental health in male and female dominated industries', *Journal of Occupational and Organisational Psychology*, Vol. 72, No. 3, pp.301-15

- Reciniello, S. (1999) 'The Emergence of a Powerful Female Workforce as a Threat to Organizational Identity', *American Behavioral Scientist*, Vol. 43, No. 2, 301-323
- Monahan, J (2001) 'The state of divorce in 21st century', *The Guardian,* 16 January 2001
- Barret, G., J. Peacock & C.R. Victor (1998) 'Are women who have abortions different from those who do not? A secondary analysis of the 1990 national survey of sexual attitudes and lifestyles', *Public Health,* Vol. 112, Issue 3, May 1998, pp 157-163
- Clarke, L., A. Berrington (1999) *'Socio-demographic predictors of divorce',* Internet www page at URL:http://www.oneplusone.org.uk/Publications/ReviewPapers/1%20-%20Socio-demographic%20predictors%20of%20divorce.pdf

CHAPTER 17 — AGEING

- Guralnik, J. M., K.C Land, D. Blazer, G.G. Fillenbaum & L.G. Branch (1993) 'Educational Status and Active Life Expectancy among Older Blacks and Whites', The New England Journal of Medicine, July 8 1993, Vol. 329, No. 2, pp 110-116
- Lin, C. C., E. Rogot, N.J. Johnson, P.D Sorlie, & E Arias (2003) 'A Further Study of Life Expectancy by Socioeconomic Factors in the National Longitudinal Mortality Study', *Ethnicity & Disease,* May 2003, Vol. 1 Issue 2, pp 240-247
- Butler, R. N, M. Fossel, S.M. Harman, C.B. Heward, S.J Olshansky, T.T Perls, D.J. Rothman, S.M. Rothman, H.R. Warner, M.D West & W.E. Wright (2002) 'Is There an Antiaging Medicine?', *The Journals of Gerontology Series A: Biological Sciences and Medical Sciences,* 2002, Vol.57, pp 333-338
- Bell, L. ed. (2007) 'Spotlight on older people in the UK', *Spotlight Report 2007*
- Department of Health, OPD(PIP) (2004) 'Better health in Old Age - Report'

- Gillmann, G., D. Harari, S. Iliffe, A.E. Stuck & C. Swift (2007) 'Health risk appraisal in older people 2: the implications for clinicians and commissioners of social isolation risk in older people', *The British Journal of General Practice*, April 1 2007, Vol. 57(537), pp 277 - 282

ABOUT PARTNERS IN MINISTRY

Partners In Ministry is a non denominational ministry that ministers through preaching, teaching, training and equipping the church to reach for spiritual revival and social reform in the nations. It carries an integrated vision to minister to the whole person, whole community and whole nation with the whole gospel. We believe strongly in the call to publication and media as a way to spread the gospel to the nations. Dr Chapman also runs biblical health and leadership seminars and conferences.

Contact details

Partners In Ministry
118 Station Road
Hendon
London
NW4 3SN
Tel: +44 (0) 208 203 9485
Email: pimchapman@aol.com

As part of this vision Dr Liam Chapman founded a charity and ministry working in northern Uganda. The East African Missionary Society has been working in an area suffering from 20 years of civil unrest. TEAMS have been working with churches establishing the Stepping Out Programme in evangelism, discipleship and leadership among men, women, youth, children and the prisons of northern Uganda. In addition it has empowered local people through orphan care, widow literacy and income generation and community development. It operates through partnership with local ministries, churches and organisations.

Contact details (address as above)

Tel: +44 (0) 208 203 5491
Website: www.teamsonline.org
Email: info@teamsonline.org

ISBN 142517627-5

9 781425 176273

Printed in Great Britain
by Amazon.co.uk, Ltd.,
Marston Gate.